AF566748

PATHS TO PSYCHIATRIC HOSPITALISATION

For Marie

Paths to Psychiatric Hospitalisation

A sociological analysis

ROGER MANKTELOW

Avebury

Aldershot · Brookfield USA · Hong Kong · Singapore · Sydney

Published by
Avebury
Ashgate Publishing Limited
Gower House
Croft Road
Aldershot
Hants GU11 3HR
England

Ashgate Publishing Company
Old Post Road
Brookfield
Vermont 05036
USA

British Library Cataloguing in Publication Data

Manktelow, Roger
Paths to Psychiatric Hospitalisation:
Sociological Analysis
I. Title
362.2
ISBN 1 85628 492 1

Library of Congress Cataloging-in-Publication Data

Manktelow, Roger 1948–
Paths to psychiatric hospitalisation : a sociological
analysis / Roger Manktelow.
p.cm.
ISBN 1-85658-492-1
1. Psychiatric hospitals--Admission and discharge--Social aspects.
2. Psychiatric hospitals--Admission and discharge--Case studies.
I. Title
RC439.M26 1994 94-9576
362.2'1--dc20 CIP

Printed and Bound in Great Britain by
Athenaeum Press Ltd, Newcastle upon Tyne.

Contents

Tables and diagrams

Acknowledgements

I would like to gratefully acknowledge the co-operation, and support of hospital and Social Services staff. I wish to record my thanks to Dr Steve Bruce and Mr Stanley Herron for their comments, guidance and advice. I wish also to thank the individuals whom as patients, clients and friends, gave me their help and co-operation and without which this research could not have been possible. Mrs Lorraine Brownlie worked hard to prepare the final manuscript and I am very grateful to her. Most of all I would like to thank my wife who has helped closely with the writing of this book.

Preface

'Our status is backed by the solid buildings of the world, while our sense of identity resides in the cracks'

Erving Goffman

'*Asylums: Essays on the Social Situations of Mental Patients and Other Inmates*' 1961, New York

Introduction

It is generally assumed that people are admitted to hospital because they are ill and that those people who are hospital patients are necessarily more ill than those outside of hospital. However, a considerable body of research in the sociology of illness shows that this is not the case and that there is a wide range of social factors outside of illness which operate to determine hospitalisation.[1] (Footnotes are at the end of the chapter). It is the purpose of this book to describe the workings of these factors in the social process of psychiatric hospitalisation. This process is enormously complicated as there is no straightforward relationship between illness and hospitalisation and, in order to make sense of it, factors other than symptomatology have to be considered. The ways in which these phenomena interact is disentangled and their operation described in the following chapters.

The field of mental illness is a quagmire for all researchers who enter it, characterised by both problems of definition and competing causal explanations. The degree of emotional commitment to and the extent of disagreement over fundamental assumptions about mental ill-health are the hallmarks of the 'paradigm clash' which Kuhn regarded as characteristic of a scientific field of enquiry in its early developmental stages.[2] How to classify the variety of human behaviour defined as abnormal is a fundamental issue. Such behaviour is characterised by Watzlawick as a circular process in which it is 'a meaningless and hopeless controversy to try to arrive at a cause'[3]. Nevertheless, a number of causal models are generally proposed, the allegiance to each being dictated as much by professional and political issues as by rational and intellectual ones.[4]

I had originally hoped in this research to provide evidence to support one such model of mental illness: the belief that mental disorder was caused by the effects of poor environment, social deprivation and social isolation. The next chapter contains such a positive-sociological approach and reports the statistical breakdown of the patient sample according to such social factors. This perspective stemmed from my own occupational experience as a social worker on an acute psychiatric ward serving an area of relative, urban deprivation.

However, it quickly became clear that it would not be possible to prove conclusively the legitimacy of one explanation over another. The theoretical issues involved are discussed in Chapter Two. At the same time, what became increasingly apparent was the crucial importance of the ways in which people became psychiatric patients and were defined as mentally ill. In Wittgenstein's words, 'our investigation is directed not towards phenomena . . . but towards the 'possibilities' of phenomena'[5]. An ethnomethodological approach is particularly suited to studying the problems of mental illness because of the disparity of behaviour subsumed under this heading. What is common is not the behaviour in all instances but the use of the concept. From this viewpoint, mental illness is described in terms of the methods and procedures which people use to describe it. This means describing how definitions and categorisations are made by individuals in an everyday manner through the use of their 'common-sense' and their 'rules of thumb'.[6]

The aim of the research is to highlight the social reality of psychiatric hospitalisation by the description of the activities of each labelling group on the route to hospital. In conclusion, a model of the hospitalisation process is tentatively proposed.

Notes

1. Susser, M. & Watson, W. ***Sociology in Medicine*** (London 1974). This book collects evidence from a large body of research in this field.
2. Kuhn, T. ***The Structure of Scientific Revolutions***, (Chicago 1962).
3. Watzlawick, P., Jackson, D. & Beavlin, J. ***Pragmatics of Human Communication***, (New York 1967).
4. Seigler, M. & Osmond, J. 'Models of Madness', ***British Journal of Psychiatry***, 112, 1966, 1193-1203. The authors identify six models: medical, moral, psychoanalytic, family-interactive, social and conspiratorial.
5. Wittgenstein, L. ***Philosophical Investigations***, (New York 1967).
6. Atkinson, M. ***Discovering Suicide. Studies in the Social Organisation of Sudden Death***, (London 1978). The author describes a similar progression in the reformulation and reinterpretation of his research.

1 Social background

In this chapter I intend to present an analysis of a group of patients admitted to psychiatric hospital over a limited period from a defined geographical area in terms of certain demographic and socio-economic factors. These variables are age, sex, marital status, living arrangement, social class, employment status, income, type of house ownership, religion and church attendance. They were selected as the most important social factors in respect of hospitalisation based on my own experience as a psychiatric social worker. The broad areas of interest and the feasibility of the study were confirmed by a pilot study in July, 1981.

The patient sample consists of all people admitted to the hospital (N = 125) over a six-month period in 1982 (from March to September), from a single local government district. For reasons elaborated below (see 'The Hospital Setting') I believe that this group represents a real measure of the use made of the psychiatric hospital by the general population from the District. A social profile of the catchment area is described in order to compare the social characteristics of the sample with the district population and to evaluate their major differences.

Such an approach is based on a positive sociological method which argues that social phenomena may be quantified and valid conclusions may be drawn from comparisons between such data. It is a major theme of this study that such exercises may not be very fruitful and that a more realistic picture is gained by the observation and description of how decisions are made and how situations are handled. The theoretical support for such a position will be outlined in the following chapter.

My own ability to follow such an approach stems from my active involvement as a member of the hospital team making decisions about patients. I was both participant and observer of the social process of psychiatric hospitalisation, and was in a position to observe and describe the ways in which members of various occupational groups, including my own, acted.

Patients were interviewed around a loose structure of open-ended questions covering biography, disturbance and the search for help. With the interviewees' permission the majority of these interviews, which ranged in duration from ten minutes to one hour, were taped. An attempt was made, where possible, to interview the patient in the first week of hospitalisation lest he be rapidly discharged (some 12% of admissions were discharged in less than one week). One advantage in getting to the patient quickly was in making the recall of events prior to hospitalisation as accurate as possible. However, the more disturbed patients could not be interviewed until their thinking had become sufficiently ordered to enable them to understand the purpose of the interview.

Only half of the sample were described diagnostically in terms of impaired thinking. Where such was the case, disturbance was compartmentalised to the extent that appropiate answers could be given about areas of everyday life. Moreover, I did not rely on a single source of information but used other sources such as case notes, the accounts of other professionals and interviews with families. Where discrepancies became evident these were often in themselves significant in indicating the values and life-styles to which people aspire.

In over 65 per cent of cases the patient was formally interviewed (N=82) and 35 per cent of these interviews were tape-recorded. Where patients were not formally interviewed there was often professional contact with the patient during ward rounds and in my daily work helping with their problems. This was supplemented by information from case notes and information gleaned from family members and other professionals. Basic demographic data was readily available from a front sheet in the case notes and circumstances of admission were detailed in the nursing cardex, the details of which could be confirmed with ward staff.

In this study the data is presented in the form of case summaries which are a synopsis of the details of each individual case. I hope that these will provide pen-pictures containing the most important aspects of the case. Inevitably, the construction of these stories is influenced by my own occupational ideology as a social worker. They are not in any sense neutral but are made up of facts which I have selected as the most important out of what may have been an amorphous body of information. The particular facts mentioned may well be different from those that would have been chosen by another occupational group but this illustrates the major contributions premise of the research that each occupational group interprets a particular situation from its own occupational perspective.

In order to unravel the social process of psychiatric hospitalisation I interviewed representatives of three occupational groups - general practitioners, clergymen and police - to investigate how they went about labelling mental illness. In my daily work as a social worker I also had the opportunity to observe how psychiatrists operated within the hospital. My work provided a unique opportunity to find out how families dealt with behaviour prior to hospitalisation. To investigate how social workers acted I analysed my own occupational activity and ideology. Each of these occupational groups are discussed in the following chapters.

The Hospital Setting

Acute psychiatric services for the catchment area of the District are divided between a psychiatric unit in a general hospital setting (suburb) and an acute admission ward in the county psychiatric hospital (New town). In an ideal situation both patient groups would be studied but concentrating on the county hospital patient group does not give rise to a skewed picture because they are similar to the patients in the general hospital.

It may be that residents of the catchment area return to hospitals in their city of origin. Hospital statistics, however, show 25 admissions to city psychiatric hospitals in 1981. (See Appendix One) Some staff believed that the more wealthy patients used the teaching hospital in the city because of its anonymity, but there was little evidence for this view. At the time of the study, the number of private psychiatrists operating was small and it was not possible to get details of their clientele. However this study is not in any sense an attempt to measure psychiatric morbidity. The county hospital patient group can, therefore, be studied as a representative sample of psychiatric hospitalisation in the District.

Prevailing ideas about in-patient psychiatric treatment hold that care in a general hospital setting is more acceptable to the public. It could, therefore, be anticipated that those most sensitive to the stigma of the mental hospital would gravitate to the general hospital setting. American research has suggested that such attitudes are more likely to be found amongst the higher social classes.[1] There was no evidence that this is the case in the present study and the social class composition of patients from the general hospital psychiatric setting were found to be similar to those entering the main psychiatric hospital. There was, however, a difference in terms of diagnoses made: those patients diagnosed as neurotic being significantly more numerous in the General Hospital Psychiatric Unit (see Appendix Two) which may be explained by the selection procedure operating in the general hospital setting. At this unit all admissions have to be first approved by the consultant and definite categories of behaviour such as alcohol abuse are excluded from admission. An alternative interpretation is that being a patient in the general setting may, of itself, help to decrease the liklihood of being given the label of a major mental illness. Furthermore the general psychiatric unit did not accept detained patients at the time of the study, which is the most likely reason for fewer psychotic patients compared to the County Hospital.

Short-term psychiatric care is provided at the county psychiatric hospital in three admission wards separately named to distance them from the stigma of the county asylum. The County Hospital was built in 1905, one of the last asylums erected in the great era of Victorian institutional provision.[2] The hospital continues to provide psychiatric in-patient beds for the whole of County (No = 300,000) At the end of the study the hospital had the lowest ratio of hospital beds to catchment population of all the Northern Ireland psychiatric hospitals.[3] This pressure on beds was an important influence on admission policy and length of stay in hospital, and particularly affected the less 'desirable' of patients.

At the time of research, compulsory admission to hospital took place under the legal framework of the 1961 Mental Health Act which has since been replaced by the 1986 Mental Health Order. This new legislation specifically excludes diagnostic categories of alcoholism and personality disorder from compulsory admission. The actual negotiation of admission usually involved a general practitioner 'requesting' a hospital bed by telephone conversation with the duty hospital doctor who would usually be his junior in terms of status. However, during regular working hours medical consultants were often available to decide on admissions. A significant number of admissions were filtered through out-patients, day-hospital and domicilary visits when a less urgent response was required. It was hospital policy for consultant approval to be sought for the admission of any person over 65 years of age. Patients were transferred from other hospitals, usually from casualty units following an overdose or other incidents of self harm and were also, exceptionally, brought directly to the hospital by the police. The whole question of pathways to hospital, a major topic in this study, will be returned to in more detail in Chapter Three.

A Social Profile of the District

The Catchment District was established in 1973 upon the reorganisation of local government. Its growth has been dependent on a population movement out of the neighbouring city. The most rapid period of growth was in the 1960's following the establishment of large factories by multi-nationals with government help. Home building took place to accommodate the new work force and the city population from slum clearance programmes.[4] Over the last 20 years the rate of population growth has slowed dramatically and has been largely unplanned and spontaneous as people sought to escape the effects of 'the Troubles'. At the 1981 census the total district population was 71,631.[5] Later population movement has been intra-district as people have moved from public to private housing which has also involved a movement up the socio-economic ladder.

The age composition of the district has altered with the slowdown in population movement: the children of those migrants of the sixties now have their own children. Three-quarters of the adult population is married; the single biggest group in the whole population is the 10-20 years age group.

The district is predominantly Protestant, and one third of the population is Presbyterian. Unemployment has increased significantly with the closure of all the multi-national factories. It stood at 11 per cent at the time of the study and has since grown substantially. In socio-economic terms the district is predominantly Social Class III which accounts for two thirds of the population.

District housing is equally divided between public and private housing with the private rented sector of minor importance.[6] The type of housing located within the three distinct areas of the district is now described.

i) Urban

The bulk of the district population, some 60,000, live in this urban area adjacent to the city boundary. It is made up of large public housing estates and private developments based on former villages. There are five public housing estates, the biggest housing 10,000 residents. The lower half of this estate has an ageing and elderly population whilst new families from the lowest social classes have moved into the top half. It is an area of social deprivation where half the children in care in the district originate and where unemployment is twice the district average. It is exclusively Protestant and significantly Church of Ireland as is a smaller but essentially similar estate. There are two newer public housing estates: which contain a pocket of social deprivation. Finally, there is a distinctive Roman Catholic area, which is historically part of the City. It, too, is an area of social deprivation with the highest rate of unemployment in the District.

The expansion of the private sector continues with home ownership falling into two broad groups. The first is a moderately priced area dominated by young families from white-collar and skilled manual occupations who are first time home buyers. This area is of mixed religious compostion. The second is a more exclusive residential area containing older housing accomodating those with professional and managerial backgrounds.

Within the urban area there are a number of garden villages, built fifty years ago to provide attractive housing at a low rent where a significant number of elderly people from professional and white collar backgrounds now reside.

ii) Market Town

This is a town of over 6,000 people serving the rural part of the district and providing some commuter accommodation. It contains a range of housing: including private building in the town environs and a pocket of social deprivation in one small public housing estate (reflected in high numbers of children in care and a high rate of unemployment).

iii) Rural

There is a large rural area of small population (5,000 people) containing a number of small villages and people, predictably, engaged in agricultural occupations. Both market town and rural hinterland are areas of strong Presbyterianism.

The Patient Sample

The patient sample consists of 125 people admitted to hospital from the catchment area over a six month period. Some people were in hospital more than once: thirteen patients were admitted twice within the survey period; four were admitted three times and one person four times. The total number of admissions in the survey period was 149. In the presentation of demographic data, statistics relate to the number of people being admitted rather than to the number of admissions, although the latter figure is used in the breakdown of routes to the hospital.

The mapping of admissions in the district was considered: locating each admission and noting clusters of admissions and relating such concentrations to the characteristics of the area. Such an approach would have followed Faris and Dunham's work in Chicago.[7] Those authors, however, used huge bodies of hospital statistics which both identified concentrations and preserved anonymity. Such an exercise was dropped from the present study because of the small number of admissions and a more interpretative approach has been emphasised.

There follows a breakdown of the patient sample according to identified social and demographic factors and a comparison with overall district proportions. The results are compared with findings from previous research. However, this is not in any sense a detailed statistical analysis. Numbers have been kept deliberately small in order to emphasise individual cases and particular instances.

The significance of social and demographic factors in mental illness has been widely investigated and a whole school of social psychiatry or psychiatric epidemiology has developed. Enormous effort and finance has been invested in the search for the 'Broad Street pump' of psychiatry.[8] In America, and to a lesser extent in Britain, whole communities have been intensively studied and some of these results are referred to. Research efforts in Ireland have naturally been less ambitious; a significant amount of research has occured abroad and been concerned with the Irish as an emigrant group in America and Britain.[9] Indigenous research has been led by the Irish Medico-Social Research Board and Dermot Walsh in particular.[10] A social anthropological approach has been followed in the intensive study of small village life in West Kerry and psychiatric hospitalisation.[11] High rates of emigration in the West of Ireland have been specifially linked to high levels of hospitalisation.[12]

Research in Northern Ireland has concentrated on the effects of the Troubles on reported mental illness. One of the effects of the early violence was found to be an increase in tranquilliser prescribing,[13] those most vulnerable being middle-aged women in urban areas and people living in areas of rural deprivation. Increased resort to the psychiatric services has been found in areas adjacent to riot areas rather than in these areas themselves.[14] Lyons argues a Durkheimian interpretation that increased opportunity to externalise aggression has led to less suffering in terms of mental health and points to the decline in the suicide rate in the early Troubles, although in recent years the rate has again risen.[15] After fifteen years of violence it may well be that a process of habituation has taken place by which people cope with the violence around them by denying its existence.[16] Northern Ireland remains an economically backward and relatively deprived area with high levels of unemployment, infant mortality, and families living below the poverty line.[17] All these factors have been identified in research elsewhere as significant influences on the level of mental illness.

Research Findings

The demographic and social variables examined divide into three groups: socio-demographic factors which have been widely investigated in hospital populations in Britain and Ireland[18]; socio-economic indicators of social deprivation which have been similarly extensively investigated; and socio-cultural factors which are more unique to the present setting. The analysis of the patient sample under investigation is presented alongside overall district figures for each variable.

i) Socio-demographic Factors

Table 1.1: Patient Sample according to Age

Age Group	Patient Sample		District Population
	Number	Per cent	over 15 years %
15-24 years	7	6.0	22.5
25-44 years	50	40.0	37.0
45-64 years	46	36.5	27.5
65-74 years	15	12.0	8.0
Over 75 years	7	5.5	5.0

The age structure of the district divides roughly into one-third under 30 years, one-third 30-50 years and one third over fifty. Given this age structure, it is clear that, as has been shown in many epidemiological surveys, the risk of hospitalisation increases with age.[19] The middle-aged are a particularly vulnerable group. It is important in any discussion to look at the ease with which different groups pass through the selection process on the way to hospital. Studies have pointed out that younger people pass through this referral process more easily than the elderly although it has been found that admission rates are much higher for the elderly group.[20] In the present sample the fact that the over-seventies are only marginally over-represented is evidence of the effectiveness of the screening procedure established to prevent elderly patients blocking acute hospital beds.

Previous research has indicated that problems with physical health are the critical antecedents to the psychiatric hospitalisation of the elderly.[21]

Table 1.2: Patient Sample according to Sex

Sex	Patient Sample		District population
	Number	Per cent	Per cent
Male	45	36.0	48.5
Female	80	64.0	51.5

In the patient sample, women outnumber men in the ratio of 3:2. This is a finding that has been confirmed in England[22] but contradicted in the Irish Republic.[23] However, in the hospital population as a whole there are more males than females. There is also evidence that the sexual ratio varies between diagnostic groups: neuroses are predominantly a female diagnosis and manic-depression is twice as frequent in females, whereas young men are the main victims of schizophrenia up to the age of thirty and alcoholism is preponderently a male diagnosis.[24]

Social epidemiological research has established that women report psychiatric symptoms more frequently than men and that their problems centre around child-management, dependent relatives, housing difficulties and marital relationships.[25]

Such problems are often greater for working class women who are also constrained from seeking help by these very problems.[26] An alternative explanation for the greater proportion of women may be that women have been socialised into seeking help.[27] In contrast, men are more likely to present with associated problems with their physical health but are also more likely to be admitted to psychiatric hospital.[28]

Table 1.3: Patient Sample According to Age and Sex.

Age group	MALE			FEMALE		
	Sample		District	Sample		District
	No.	%	%	No.	%	%
15-24 yrs	4	8.0	24.0	4	4.5	21.5
25-44 yrs	24	52.0	38.0	27	33.5	36.0
45-64 yrs	10	25.0	28.0	34	43.0	27.5
65-74 yrs	5	11.0	7.0	10	13.0	9.0
Over 75	2	4.0	3.0	5	6.0	6.0

It can be seen that men are most at risk of psychiatric hospitalisation at a younger age than women, being most over-represented in the age range 25-44 years. In contrast, women enter hospital most frequently in middle-age, as shown by their over-representation in the 45-64 years age group. This fact, which has been widely found, has been explained in terms of middle-age being a transitional stage for women when they are experiencing significant (menopausal) physical changes and role changes (when their children are becoming independent) which leave them vulnerable to emotional breakdown.

As expected from previous research, the likelihood of psychiatric admission increases with age, and both sexes are over represented in the elderly group. Elderly women, however, enter hospital in greater numbers than men, which may well be a reflection of their greater life-expectancy. Such results have been reported in British epidemiological studies and summarised as follows: more men than women being admitted under 25; women being more numerous over 25 years, particularly in middle-age; and male rates rising again after middle-age but still remaining lower than female.[29]

Table 1.4: Patient Sample according to Marital Status

Marital status	Patient Sample Number	Patient Sample %	District %
Single	29	23.5	15.5
Married/Cohabitating	55	44.0	75.0
Widowed	15	12.0	8.0
Separated/Divorced	26	20.5	(1.5) div.

There are clear differences in marital status in the patient sample as compared with the district population. A much lower proportion of people admitted to hospital are married and an equivalently larger proportion are single, widowed or separated. The percentage separated or divorced is significantly higher but the district figure only indicates divorced persons. Marriage breakdown is clearly associated with hospitalisation although it is not clear whether it results from the existence of psychiatric disorder or acts as a precipitant to breakdown.

Marital status is a powerful factor in psychiatric hospitalisation rates. The risk of entry to psychiatric treatment rises in a gradient from the married, through the single to the widowed and separated and divorced.[30] However, it is not clear to what extent it is cause or consequence.

Clearly, people suffering mental disorder are less likely to be married, being less able to cope with the demands of sustaining a close, emotional relationship. This may be part of the reason for prolonged bachelorhood as in the West of Ireland where 80 per cent of hospital patients are unmarried.[31]

This means missing out on the primary social arrangement for intimate support available in our society. Marriage can help people fend off the psychological assaults that economic and social problems create. There is evidence that when one is confronted with these strains and is single, then one is more prone to depression.[32] But it is the quality of relationship which is important as was illustrated by the working class women of Camberwell. Those who were without an intimate relationship with their husband/boyfriend were more vulnerable to depression.[33] The status transition to widowhood, separation or divorce leaves the individual more vulnerable to psychiatric breakdown particularly in the short-term.[34]

Table 1.5: Patient Sample according to Marital Status and Sex

Marital status	MALE			FEMALE		
	Patient Sample		District Pop.	Patient Sample		District Pop.
	No.	%	%	No.	%	%
Single	17	37.5	17.0	12	15.5	14.0
Married/ Cohabitating	23	52.0	78.0	31	39.0	72.0
Widowed	1	2.0	3.0	14	18.0	12.0
Separated/ Divorced	4	8.5	1.0	23	27.5	1.5 (div)

An analysis by marital status and sex shows up important differences between males and females. Firstly, a much higher proportion of men admitted are single which would seem to suggest that marriage offers greater protection of mental health for men than women. This view is supported by the evidence that when marital breakdown occurs it is the separated wife who is more likely to end up in psychiatric hospital. There may be several reasons for this: in the first place, women are much more likely to be widowed than men and this is reflected in the considerably larger numbers of widows being admitted to hospital; in the second place it seems likely that when marriages break down it is women who are most likely to be left to care for the children and face the financial and housing problems which add up to significant life event stresses.

There would seem to be two particular groups at risk of hospitalisation. Firstly, bearing in mind the very small numbers of men under 25 years admitted, there would appear to be a group of men who do not marry and who appear vulnerable to psychiatric disorder. Secondly, and in contrast, for women it is marital breakdown, whether through death or separation, that is the most important factor in female hospitalisation, being present in nearly half of female admissions. These findings correspond with other research which has reported the highest rates of hospitalisation amongst single men and divorced persons of both sexes.[35]

The variables identified serve as indicators of characteristics of patients' lives and these variables interact in particular ways. Having sketched the demographic features of the patient population in terms of sex, age and marital status, I will now examine social deprivation.

ii) Socio-Economic Factors

It has been widely found that mental disorders are concentrated in the poorest classes: some twenty eight studies have shown an association between low socio-economic status and high rates of mental disorder.[36] Psychiatric hospitalisation is significantly a lower-class experience.[37] In England, the highest rates of hospital admissions have been found amongst labourers and kitchen hands,[38] whilst in Ireland, agricultural workers have, by far, the highest rate of hospitalisation.[39] Social deprivation is particularly concentrated in inner city areas where high rates of psychiatric hospitalisation are found.[40] For instance, in the London Borough of Camden it was found that of their psychiatric patients on one day, 28 per cent came from transitory accommodation and 64 per cent were unemployed.[41] I will now describe a number of indicators of socio-economic status.

Table 1.6: Patient Sample according to Social Class

Social class	Patient Sample		District Population
	Number	Per cent	Per cent
S.C.I	1	1	3.5
S.C.II	10	8	14.0
S.C.III	52	41	63.5
S.C.IV.	46	37	13.5
S.C.V.	16	12	5.5

Whilst the catchment area is predominantly working class, psychiatric hospitalisation is overwhelmingly a lower social class experience. In the sample, there are nearly three times as many patients in Social Class IV as in the district population. If S.C.III (skilled and clerical workers), S.C.IV (the semi-skilled), and S.C.V (the unskilled) are grouped together to form the working class, then this group accounts for 91 per cent of admissions. There are a number of explanations for this preponderance of working class patients.The breeder or social drift hypothesis emphasises hereditary factors and the drift down the social scale of handicapped individuals as explanation.[42] In the present study, there was only marginal evidence of a social drift between S.C.IV and S.C.V. Social causation theorists, on the other hand, emphasise the effects of poverty, poor housing and hardship in causing mental breakdown.[43]

Social class is an important determinant of the threshhold for seeking psychiatric help. In America, the expectation of the lower class that, should they seek psychiatric help, they will be incarcerated in a state asylum makes for a delay in seeking psychiatric treatment.[44] In the Camberwell study it was found that the social factors that make the working class woman more vulnerable to depression also act as a barrier to seeking psychiatric care.[45] Studies of social class habits of consulting in the National Health Service have suggested that, whilst the lower social classes make heavier demands for consultations,[46] they, relatively, underuse facilities associated with prevention.[47]

When other factors are taken into account with social class, particular groups have been identified as being vulnerable to psychiatric hositalisation. For instance, it has been found that a single person from S.C.V. is thirty times more likely than a married person from S.C.I. to be admitted to psychiatric hospital.[48] If diagnostic grouping is taken into consideration it seems that some types of mental disorder, principally schizophrenia, contribute to the excess in the lower social classes. It has been found that schizophrenia is eleven times more frequent in S.C.V than in S.C.I., whilst affective disorders are more evenly spread throughout the classes.[49] Neurotic patients from the lower social classes have been found to be 'sicker' in terms of their symptoms than upper class neurotic patients, which may be caused by the more serious social problems of bad housing and low income found amongst the lower class patients.[50]

Finally, it has been found that suicide is related to poverty and unemployment when other factors of social disorganisation are present.[51]

Table 1.7: Patient Sample according to Employment Status

Employment Status	Patient Sample Number	Patient Sample Per cent		District Per cent
Employed	19	15		59
Unemployed	28	22		6
Retired	31	25		10
Student/sheltered	1	1		5
Husband employed	18	14)		
Housewife/ Single parent	11	9)	37	20% (inactive)
Unfit for work	17	14)		

The level of unemployment in the patient group was over three times higher than the district average, whilst the number of patients who were working, or whose spouses were in employment was only half the district figure. This is a clear indicator of deprivation being experienced by patients and their families. In total some 85 per cent of the people coming into hospital were not working; such a major proportion cannot simply be explained by the disabling effect of the onset of psychiatric disturbance. Within this figure are a quarter of the sample who are retired and who are significantly over- represented, a reflection of the increased rate of hospitalisation for the elderly.

These findings are broadly in agreement with previous research which on a macro-level has related increases in unemployment to increased rates of hospitalisation.[52] Small scale studies have, however, emphasised the importance of group membership as a buffer to the psychological depression of redundancy.[53] The effects of unemployment in Hartlepool were mediated through a deterioration in personal relationships which may act as a catalyst to para-suicide.[54]

Finally, George Brown's study emphasised the lack of full-time or part-time work as a vulnerability factor increasing the likelihood of depression.[55]

Table 1.8: Patient Sample according to Type of Income

Income	Patient Sample	
	Number	Per cent
Wages	32	26
Retirement pension	34	27
Invalidity benefit	19	15
Other statutory benefit	12	10
Supplementary benefit	28	22

It can be seen that some three quarters of the patient sample are dependent on some form of state benefit. This figure, together with the previously found high level of economic inactivity are strong indicators of a high level of material and social deprivation found in the study. This is further emphasised by the fact that some 22 per cent of the sample were wholly dependent on supplementary benefit (now Income Support). Supplementary benefit is paid at subsistence level. It may, therefore, be said that over a fifth of patients coming into hospital were living in poverty. In the sample as a whole there were, in fact, more people living on retirement pension than in receipt of a wage income. This finding reflects the elderly bias in the patient sample but, nevertheless, it is an extraordinary result.

Table 1.9: Patient sample according to Type of Housing

Housing	Patient Sample		District[56]
	Number	Per cent	%
N.I.H.E.(public)	75	60	44.0
Owner occupied	30	24	45.0
Private rented	12	9	9.5
Sheltered accommodation	6	5	1.5
No fixed abode	2	1	-

House ownership may be viewed as a measure of social status; conversely, renting your home may be an indicator of relative deprivation. In the district as a whole, the proportion of public housing and owner occupied are similar.

However, in the patient sample those living in public housing are over-represented whilst those owning their homes are under-represented. This finding may be interpreted as an indicator of relative deprivation amongst those entering psychiatric hospital. The proportion from private rented accommodation reflects the district average whilst the number of no fixed abode is insignificant.

Past research has been based on the expectation that improvements in the social environment, such as better housing and planned communities, would bring about improvements in mental health. However, it has been found that a post-war new housing estate outside London had a relatively high incidence of psychological disorder.[57] Similarly, the investigation of a planned new town found a higher rate of reported neurotic disorder than the national average.[58] The authors explained this finding by a lowering of the threshhold for reporting symptoms to the doctor which was largely attributed to the establishment of new health centres with doctors eager to build up practices. Living in high and low-rise flats has been investigated and found to be associated with an increased reporting of depression and loneliness for young mothers as compared with those living in more conventional housing.[59]

Taken together, the four variables of social class composition, unemployment, dependence on statutory benefit and public housing all point to a high level of social deprivation in the patient sample. How this may be interpreted is a subject of theoretical discussion in the next chapter. For the moment, it may suffice to say that, whilst it cannot be categorically stated that poverty causes mental illness, nor that mental illness causes poverty, it is clear that deprivation, both real and relative, is a factor in the life- situations of a considerable number of people coming into hospital.

iii) Socio-Cultural Factors

Subsumed under this heading are those factors that indicate the chief cultural characteristics of the patient sample, in particular religious affiliation. There is also some attempt to measure in quantitatative terms the level of social disintegration and social isolation. It is a fundamental proposition of Durkheimian sociology that such factors are crucial explanations of psychological phenomena, specifically suicide.[60] One of the chief measures of such disintegration in a religious society is the level of church attendance, which will be examined. Attention has also been particularly concentrated on social isolation as a causal explanation of mental disorder.[61] However, recent research has recognised the need for some qualitative measure of social interaction to supplement a quantitative approach.[62] In the present study, attempts to measure the extent and content of social networks as well as 'an Index of Leisure Activity'[63] were abandoned due to insufficient time and resources.

Table 1.10: Patient Sample according to Living Arrangement

Living arrangement	Patient Number	Sample %	District %
Alone	34	27.0	5
With spouse	22	18.0	14.5
With siblings	4		
With parents	14	16.5	
With adult children	3		69.0*
Parenting	31	25.0	
Single parent	9	7.0	8*
Sheltered accommodation	6	4.5	0.5
No fixed abode	2	2.0	-

* District figures include non-dependent children with no age limits.

Most strikingly, it can be seen that those living alone are disproportionately represented in the patient group, being five times more numerous than in the district as a whole. This relationship between social isolation and psychiatric hospitalisation has been widely established in a variety of areas. It was first recognised in Chicago where there was a concentration of schizophrenics in rooming house districts,[64] and later confirmed in nine other American cities,[65] at least one American state[66], and in the English city of Bristol.[67]

Although the results are difficult to interpret it seems that those looking after children were less likely to be admitted to hospital. The district figures, however, do not differentiate between adult and young children so that elderly parents living with their grown-up children are included in this group. It may well be that single parents are over- represented, as would be anticipated from the Camberwell study. The situation may be clarified when living arrangement is next analysed according to sex.

Table 1.11: The Patient Sample according to Living Arrangement and Sex

Living arrangement	Patient Sample			
	MALE		FEMALE	
	Number	%	Number	%
Living alone	9	21.0	25	31.0
With spouse	9	19.0	14	18.0
With Sibling	2		2	
With parents	8	23.0	5	13.0
With grown-up children	-		3	
Parenting	14	31.0	17	21.5
Single parenting	-	-	9	11.0
Sheltered accommodation	2	4.0	4	4.5
No fixed abode	1	2.0	1	1.0

The table shows a different picture for each sex. For males, 37% of whom have already been found to be single, a considerable proportion live alone but, more significantly, nearly as many live at home with their parents. This would seem to indicate a group of single men at home who have not achieved independence and who are vulnerable to psychiatric hospitalisation. On the other hand, for women nearly a third of the sample live alone and this proportion may be explained by the greater numbers of widowed and elderly females. When the parenting group is examined according to sex, it is clear that men are more frequently admitted to hospital than their spouses. This may well be because of the greater importance of women in the family in their mothering and caring role, a role which leaves them less able to resort to psychiatric hospitalisation. The fact that all single parents admitted to hospital are female points up the possibility that these women have been left to shoulder child-care and financial responsibilities on their own which have overwhelmed them.

Table 1.12: Patient Sample according to Mobility

Length of occupation	Patient Sample	
	Number	Per cent
Under 2 years	21	16.5
2 - 5 years	21	16.5
5 - 10 years	26	21.0
10 years and over	40	32.0
Not known	17	14.0

The catchment area is predominantly stable and the largest group are those in residence for over ten years. The figures are difficult to interpret because of the absence of district figures for comparison but it is worth noting that nearly a sixth of the sample have moved within the last two years.

Previous research has found that high mobility is a significant factor in relation to the level of psychiatric illness in general practice;[68] in the number of psychiatric admissions from London Boroughs[69] and the number of suicides[70].

Table 1.13: Patient Sample according to Religious Affiliation

Church	Patient Sample		District
	Number	%	%
Protestant:			
Church of Ireland	44	35.5	23.0
Presbyterian	33	26.5	33.5
Non-conformist	13	10.0	13.0
Evangelical	17	13.5	3.0
Roman Catholic	18	14.5	8.5
Not stated	-	-	18.0

In Northern Ireland, religious affiliation is of crucial importance and social significance. The relationship between religious affiliation and two particular psychiatric diagnoses of schizophrenia and alcoholism has been investigated elsewhere.[71] The authors found that Catholics were more likely to be hospitalised than Protestants but suggested there were two distinct groups of patients according to area of origin. These were 'West of the Bann', Catholic, rural, bachelor, male patients (essentially similar to the patients of the West of Ireland), with high rates of admission, and a second distinctive group in the industrial East, which was predominantly Protestant with fewer admissions and a prevalence similar to that found in England.[72]

Interpretation of the present findings is made difficult by the high percentage of 'not stated' reported in the 1981 Census. A similar response in 1971 prompted the calculation that 15 per cent of Catholics did not answer the religious question as compared with 6 per cent of Protestants.[73] Taking this into account and the fact that church membership is related to social class in the district, some tentative interpretations are made. The over-representation of Church of Ireland members who are located in the public housing estates, is related to the preponderance of the lower social classes in the patient sample. The converse is true for the under representation of the Presbyterian group who are concentrated in the rural areas of the district. The non-conformist churches are made up of the Congregational, Methodist and Baptist churches and are also slightly under-represented. Catholics are somewhat over-represented although it is difficult to make an accurate comparison because of the level of non-response to the religious question in the General Census. Most dramatic is the relatively large number of evangelical church members which may be explained by the particularly heavy demands associated with church membership.

Table 1.14: Patient Sample according to Church Attendance

Attendance	Patient Sample	
	Number	Per cent
Attending	36	29
Non-attending	70	56
Not known	19	15

The fairly high non-return rate makes it difficult to interpret the figures but an inevitable conclusion is that church affiliation is nominal in many cases.

Table 1.15: Patient Sample according to Religious Affiliation and Church Attendance

	Patient Sample				
/Church Attendance	C. of I.	Presbyt.	Non-Con.	Evang.	R.C.
Attending	3	7	4	10	13
Non-attending	29	24	8	6	3
Not known	12	2	1	1	3
Total	44	33	13	17	18

With the usual rider about non-return, some wide variations are immediately apparent. The extremely low involvement in the Church of Ireland may be explained by the nominal nature of C. of I. membership as compared to the evangelical group or the Catholic Church. However, it is an extremely low figure. The Presbyterians also have a low level of church attendance which is unusual, bearing in mind the existence in rural areas of established families with strong traditions of church-going. In the case of the main Protestant churches hospitalisation is associated with low levels of attendance. But the relationship is reversed for evangelicals.

These churches demand a high level of social, spiritual and sometimes financial commitment and it is the extent of this commitment that may become a source of stress to the member concerned. Finally, the level of church attendance for the Catholic group is high, reflecting the pattern of high attendance found in the Catholic Church overall and the requirement on the individual to perform spiritual duties.

This section has attempted to establish some aspects of the socio-cultural context of the patient sample. In broad terms evidence has been produced of a degree of social isolation, a small measure of geographical mobility and some social disintegration in terms of a breakdown in traditional patterns of church going.

Summary

This chapter has considered the relevance of age, sex, marital status, social class, employment status, income, housing, living arrangement, mobility, and religious affiliation to admissions to psychiatric hospital. People admitted are, on the whole, older, more likely to be women, be unmarried, living alone, working class, unemployed, dependent on state benefit, living in public housing, to have lived there for some time and are less likely to attend church. The broad picture is therefore of a deprived group of people in terms of social disintegration, employment, income and housing as compared with the population at large. Within this generalisation there is also evidence of vulnerable sub- groups: single men over the age of 25 still living with their parents; widows over the age of 45; and young women who are legally separated and who are single parents.

The next chapter is concerned with the question to what extent various interpretations of the data are valid and definitive and finding the most useful and appropiate method of investigating the social aspects of the process of psychiatric hospitalisation.

Notes

1. Hollingshead, A. and Redlich, F. (1958) *Social Class and Mental Ilness.* This study showed a marked reluctance for higher social class persons to enter the state psychiatric hospital. New York.
2. Finnane, M. (1981) *Insanity and the Insane in Post-Famine Ireland.* Croom Helm.
3. Department of Health and Social Services, (1979) *Psychiatric Hospitals in Northern Ireland: A Survey of Physical Facilities and Estimate of Future Needs.*
4. O'Dowd, L., Rolston, B. and Tomlinson, M. (1980) *Northern Ireland: Between Civil Rights and Civil War* Brandon.
5. *Official Census of Northern Ireland 1981.*
6. Northern Ireland Housing Executive, (1979) *Home Condition Survey.*
7. Faris, R. and Dunham, H. (1939) *Mental Disorders in Urban Areas*, Chicago.
8. Strauss, J. (1979) 'Social and Cultural Influences on Psychopathology', *Psychological Annual Review*, 30, pp. 397-415.
   Wankin, J., Fleming, D., Buck, C. and Hobbs, G. (1955) 'Factors influencing the Rate of First Admissions to Mental hospital', *Journal of Nervous and Mental Disease*, 121, pp. 103-16.
9. Cochrane, R. and Stopes-Roe, M. (1979) 'Psychological disturbance in Ireland, in England and in Irish Emigrants to England: a Comparative Study.' *Economic and Social Review*, 10, pp. 301-20.
10. Walsh, D., and O'Hare, A. (1981) *The Third Census of Irish Psychiatric Hospitals*. The Medico-Social Research Board, Dublin.
11. Scheper-Hughes, N. (1979) *Saints, Scholars and Schizophrenics - Mental Illness in Rural Ireland.* Los Angeles.
12. Walsh, D. (1969) 'Two and Two makes Five: Multifactorigenesis in Mental Illness in Ireland', *Journal of Irish Medical Association*, 69, pp. 417-422.
13. Frazer, R. (1971) 'The Cost of Commotion: An Analysis of the Psychiatric Sequelae of the 1969 Riots'. *British Journal of Psychiatry*, 118, pp. 257-64.
    King, D., Griffiths, K. and Merret, J. 'Psychotropic Drug Use in Northern Ireland 1966-1980'. *Psychological Medicine*, 12, pp. 819-32.

14. Lyons, H. (1972) 'Depressive Illness and Aggression in Belfast', *British Medical Journal.*
15. Moloney, E. (1983) 'Suicides and The New Normality' *Irish Times* March 12, 1983.
16. Cairns, E. and Wilson, R. (1984) 'The Impact of Political Violence on Mild Psychiatric Morbidity in Northern Ireland', *British Journal of Psychiatry*, 145.
17. Evason, E. (1980) 'Ends that won't meet: A Study of Poverty in Belfast', *CPAG Poverty Research Series*, No. 8.
18. Hammond, A. (1970) 'An Analysis of Psychiatric Hospital Admissions for the London Boroughs, 1966', *Greater London Intelligence Unit Quarterly Bulletin*, 12, pp. 23-9.
19. Innes, G. and Sharpe, G. (1962) 'A Study of Psychiatric Patients in North-East Scotland', *Journal of Mental Science*, 108, pp.447-56.
    Adelstein, A., Downham, D., Stein, Z. and Susser, M. (1968) 'The Epidemiology of Mental Illness in an English City Salford', *Social Psychiatry*, 3, pp. 47-59.
20. Roberson, M. (1979) 'Variations in Referral Patterns to the Psychiatric Services by General Practitioners', *Psychological Medicine*, 9, pp. 355-64.
21. Lowenthal, M. (1964) 'Social Isolation and Mental Ilness in Old Age', *American Sociological Review*, pp. 54-70.
22. Carstairs, G., Tonge, W., O'Connor, J. and Barber, L. (1955) 'Changing Population of Mental Hospitals', *British Journal of Preventative Social Medicine*, 9, pp. 187-90.
23. Walsh, D. (1968) 'Mental Illness in Dublin: First Admissions', *British Journal of Psychiatry*, 114, pp. 11-14.
24. Ibid.
25. Shepherd, M. (1966) *Psychiatric Illness in General Practice*, Oxford.
26. Brown, G. and Harris, T. (1978) *Social Origins of Depression*. London.
27. Philips, D. and Segal, B. (1969) 'Sexual Status and Psychiatric Symptoms', *American Sociological Review*, 29, pp. 679-87.
28. Hopkins, P. and Cooper, B. (1969) 'Psychiatric Referral from General Practice', *British Journal of Psychiatry*, 115, pp. 1163-74.
29. Adelstein et al (1968) op. cit.
30. Ibid.
31. Walsh, D. and O'Hare, A. (1983) *Activities of Irish Psychiatric Hospitals and Units. 1980.* Dublin.
32. Pearlin, L. and Johnson, J. (1977) 'Marital Status, Life-strains and Depression', *Americal Sociologial Review*, 42, pp. 104-15.
33. Brown, G. (1978), op. cit.
34. Stein, Z. and Susser, M. (1969), op. cit.
35. Adelstein, A. et al (1968), op. cit.
36. Dohrenwend, B. and Dohrenwend, B.S. (1974) 'Social and Cultural Influences on Pathology', *Annual Review of Psychology*, 25, pp. 417-52.
37. Hollingshead, A. and Redlich, F. (1958), op. cit.
38. Brooke, E. (1959) 'National Studies in the Epidemiology of Mental Illness', 105, pp. 803-908.
39. Walsh, D. and O'Hare, A. (1983), op. cit.
40. Faris, R. and Dunham, H. (1930), op. cit.

41. Ebringer, L. and Christe-Brown, J. (1980) 'Social Deprivation amongst Short-Stay Psychiatric Patients', *British Journal of Psychiatry*, 16, pp. 46-52.
42. Goldberg, E. and Morrison, S. (1963) 'Schizophrenia and Social Class', *British Journal of Psychiatry*, 109, pp. 785-802.
43. Brown, G. and Harris, T. (1978), op. cit.
44. Hollingshead, A. and Redlich, F. (1958), op. cit.
45. Brown, G. and Harris, T. (1978), op. cit.
46. Kedward, H. (1962) 'Social Habits of Counselling', *British Journal of Preventative Social Medicine*, 16, pp. 147-52.
47. Alderson, M. (1970) 'Social Class and the Health Service', *The Medical Officer*, 17 July 1970, pp. 50-52.
48. Brooke, E. (1959), op. cit.
49. Hollingshead, A. and Redlich, F. (1958), op. cit.
50. Kedward, H. (1969) 'The Outcome of Neurotic Illness in the Community', *Social Psychiatry*, 4, pp. 1-4.
51. Sainsbury, P. (1955) *Suicide in London: an Ecological Study*, Maudsley Monographs No. 1. London.
52. Brenner, H. (1973) *Mental Ilness and the Economy* Harvard.
53. Figueria-McDonagh, J. (1978) 'Mental Health among Unemployed Detroiters', *Social Services Review.*
54. Furness, J., Khan, M. and Pickens, P. (1985) 'Unemployment and Para-suicide in Hartlepool, 1974-83', *Health Trends*, 17, pp. 21-24.
55. Brown, G. and Harris, T. (1978), op. cit.
56. Northern Ireland Housing Executive (1979), op. cit.
57. Martin, F., Brotherston, J. and Chave, S. (1957) 'Incidence of Neurosis in a New Housing Estate', *British Journal of Preventative Social Medicine*, 11, pp. 196-202.
58. Taylor, L. and Chave, S. (1964) *Mental Health and the Environment*, London.
59. Richman, N. (1974) 'The Effects of Housing on Pre-school Children and their Mothers', *Developmental Medical Child Neurology*, 16, pp. 53-58.
60. Durkheim, E. (1951) *Suicide: A Study in Sociology*, Glencoe.
61. Faris, R. and Dunham, H. (1939), op. cit.
62. Gottlieb, B. (1983) *Social Networks and Social Supports*, New York.
63. Taylor, L. and Chave, S. (1964), op. cit.
64. Faris, R. and Dunham, H. (1939), op. cit.
65. Clarke, R. (1949) 'Psychoses, Income and Occupational Prestige: Schizophrenia in American Cities', *American Journal of Sociology*, 54, pp. 433-40.
66. Jaco, E. (1960) The Social Epidemiology of Mental Disorders: *A Psychiatric Survey of Texas*, New York.
67. Hare, E. (1956) 'Mental Illness and Social Conditions in Bristol', *Journal of Mental Science*, 102, pp. 349-57.
68. Shepherd, M. (1966), op. cit.
69. Hammond, A. (1970), op. cit.
70. Sainsbury, P. (1955), op. cit.
71. Murphy, H. (1975) 'Alcoholism and Schizophrenia in the Irish: A Review'. *Transcultural Psychiatric Research Review*, 12, pp. 116-39.

72. Murphy, H. and Vega, G. (1982) 'Schizophrenia and Religious Affiliation in Northern Ireland', *Psychological Medicine*, pp. 595-605.
73. Compton, P. As quoted in the Belfast Telegraph, 21st January 1983.

2 Theoretical issues

The breakdown of the patient sample has revealed a group of people who are deprived both economically and socially. Their main social characteristics are low class, low income, unemployment, and living in public housing with some social isolation. These findings are now discussed in terms of the main ideological perspectives operating in the field of mental illness. On the basis of this discussion I will argue that the process of psychiatric hospitalisation can best be conceptualised by a perspective that includes labelling theory and the ethnomethodological approach.

The medical model explains the apparent class dimension of psychiatric hospital admissions by supposing that the causes of mental illness, which it locates in the individual, are genetically transmitted. This 'breeder' hypothesis supposes that a predisposition to psychiatric problems becomes predominant in one class rather than another because both class position and a tendency to mental illness are transmitted by genetic inheritance.[1]

The etiology of mental illness is described as an imbalance in brain biochemistry and the lower classes are assumed to suffer disproportionately. Enormous research effort has been expended in the search to identify this etiological process but the evidence remains largely speculative.[2]

Another explanation put forward by psychiatrists is the social drift hypothesis which argues that handicapped people and social failures drift down the social scale because of the disabling effects of their psychiatric condition.[3] Evidence has been produced that the fathers of patients have a higher occupational status than their children and that the occupational history of patients themselves shows a downward drift.[4] Other researchers have argued against such findings and in the present study, there is only marginal evidence of social drift and it is confined to the lower occupational strata.

The psychological perspective explains the preponderance of the lower social classes in psychiatric hospital by their lack of ego strengh which is blamed on early child-rearing practices. It is argued that these practices produce personalities which are physically aggressive, dependent on others and which require immediate tangible rewards.[6] Amongst the lower social classes there is also a greater experience of family disruption and more likelihood of removal into a children's home with consequent long-term adverse psychological effects.[7] The solution for such troubles is psychoanalysis or psychotherapy. However, lower class people are unlikely to be motivated towards seeking such help and, more importantly, unable to afford it. Is it possible, then, that all the middle class individuals with psychiatric problems are receiving such treatment and, thereby, avoiding coming into hospital? There is little evidence to support such an interpretation: G.P.s reported few cases of people requesting such help and there was no evidence of middle class patients from the district using one possible source of such therapy, the Professorial Psychiatric Unit in the nearby city.[8]

The social-psychiatrist explains the high numbers of working-class patients in terms of their greater endurance of social stressors which precipitate breakdown. George Brown argues that not only do working class women experience more loss and threat of loss, as well as more long-term difficuties, but they are also, more often, less equipped to resolve such problems because of their social isolation.[9] However, some researchers argue that such psychiatric disorders are transitory and do not require further referral or hospitalisation.[10] There is clearly a difference of opinion here in what constitutes a psychiatric case and the root problems of definition are discussed fully below.

The combination of psychiatry and sociology into social psychiatry has been something of an unholy alliance in which strains become evident with the consideration of the power dimension in psychiatric hospitalisation.[11] The use of power is determined by material resources and membership of a dominant culture. Sociological explanations of the class bias found amongst psychiatric patients have concentrated on the link between deprivation, an indicator of the absence of power, and psychiatric hospitalisation. Such studies are firmly rooted within the positivist tradition of sociology.[12]; the fact that lower class patients predominate has been explained by their poor material circumstances.[13] A similarly striking finding of an over-proportion of lower class patients has been found for chronic sickness and infant mortality.[14]

Sociologists have also proposed a cultural explanation which argues that the values of a particular class sub-culture determine access to technical knowledge and specialised services.The lower social classes are believed to have a more fatalistic attitude towards life, attributing troubles to unhappiness, bad luck or physical illness rather than psychogenic factors.[15] Moreover, their experience and knowledge of the way in which the psychiatric services work (long-term hospitalisation and physical methods of treatment) are likely to lead them to delay seeking psychiatric help for as long as possible.[16] Some researchers attribute long-term hospitalisation to this delay.[17] On the other hand, the same hospital data has been interpreted as evidence that lower class persons are admitted more often because of their lack of power.[18] Finally, a further interpretation that has been proposed is that middle class individuals seek psychiatric help quicker because of their greater significance and importance which means filling more roles and, therefore, having greater visibility.[19]

The middle classes may also use their resources to avoid the stigmatising label of mental illness by being treated in general hospital for physical illness and by resisting efforts to reinterpret their symptoms as mental illness. They are also likely to have more alternative and less stigmatising forms of deviance available to them. Some of these alternatives may be in the nature of 'escape attempts' from everyday life such as holidays abroad, expensive hobbies and encounter groups.[20] Whilst lower class people may have similar needs to escape the pressures of everyday life, their opportunities to do so may be restricted to T.V. soap operas, the betting shop and drunken oblivion. Moreover, their efforts to 'escape' as football hooligan, welfare scrounger and telephone vandal, are, themselves, likely to bring them into conflict with authority. The lower class person is therefore much more likely to infringe social values and be labelled deviant, an occasion of itself which gives an opportunity for social norms and rules to be reaffirmed.[21]

If we suppose that the support of primary networks gives some protection against mental illness[22], the absence of such support - social isolation - should be linked to the appearance of psychiatric problems, and it has been argued that social isolation is characteristic of the lowest social strata.[23] Faris and Dunham explain the concentration of paranoid schizophrenics in rooming houses in Chicago by the absence of healthy communication against the disorganised environment of the inner city which leads to mental breakdown.[24] The fact that rates of psychiatric hospitalisation are highest in these city-centre districts which also have the highest rates of delinquency, crime, mortality, poverty and unemployment, has resulted in social disintegration being put forward as an explanation of mental illness.[25] Smaller disintegrated rural communities have also been identified as causing 'malfunctioning personalities'.[26]

The fundamental problem that besets all these interpretations is that it is difficult to know which is the independent variable and which is the dependent variable in the relationship. For instance, does the poverty and stress of lower class living cause schizophrenia or does the disabling effects of the condition result in movement down the social scale? Similarly, does living alone in a lodging house cut off from human contact cause schizophrenic breakdown, or do schizophrenics end up in such twilight zones because of the isolating effects of their illness? Part of the difficulty of interpretation stems from the fact that such variables are themselves taken into consideration in the process of definition. In other words, living alone and low social class are both likely to be factors that are called upon as evidence (amongst other variables) to support the definition of illness. This issue is addressed by Atkinson in his study of suicide in which he quotes Blum and McHugh's description of killing oneself as a method of doing depression in the same way as prematurely leaving the party is a way of doing boredom.[27]

It can be seen that any interpretation of the proponderence of the lower class in the patient sample has a strong ideological component.[28] From this standpoint, the fact of hospitalisation may be viewed as a reflection of the ideologies of the actors and agents involved in the process. Hospital admission statistics provide information about people's preparedness to use medical forms of care and accept medical interpretations of their behaviour.[28] However, they are also official statistics and as such may say more about the ideologies and methodologies of the personnel whose responsibility it is to collect them.[29] It has been argued that such official rates tell us more about organisational processes than about the incidence of forms of behaviour.[30] Moreover, the low priority given by hospital administrative procedures to the collection of hospital statistics has important implications for the reliability of such data.[31]

Much epidemiological effort has been invested by psychiatrists in the investigation of the 'real' rate of mental illness. Communities have been trawled to discover this 'true incidence' but such studies have produced a wide variety of results.[32] Such findings are a reflection of the methods used: hospital statistics report the lowest level of mental illness; community surveys find more cases from G.P.s and other records; and direct interviews with a sample of the general population find the highest level.[33] As Taylor and Chave state: 'the size of the catch depends on the size of the mesh of the net used'.[34] Psychiatrists can be seen to differ in their definition of what constitutes mental illness and the over-enthusiastic diagnostician can find evidence of mental ill-health in most human beings.[35]

What is of importance is the way in which definitions are applied, which is not done so much by psychiatrists as individuals outside hospital. People arrive in hospital on the basis of lay definitions of their behaviour; lay members make ascriptions on the basis of 'untechnical' common sense competence and the professional uses his competence to ratify these ascriptions. In the normal run of events, the fact of hospitalisation is accepted as evidence of illness. It is this process of definition that requires investigation. Otherwise, as has been shown in the previous discussion, any attempt to explain mental illness in terms of extrinsic factors such as social class leads to circular arguments. Moreover, any attempts to seek a 'real' measure of mental illness results in wide disagreement over what constitutes such a phenomena. We are left with describing the phenomenon of mental illness in terms of the way in which the concept is employed, the evidence of its use being shown in the fact of hospitalisation.

Theoretical support for such an approach is provided by the labelling perspective as elaborated in respect of mental illness by Thomas Scheff.[37] Scheff argues that such is the diversity of behaviour which is included under the rubric of mental illness that it resists distillation into common characteristics. He explains this diversity in terms of the use of the label of mental illness as a residual category within which are lumped together 'the most diverse kinds of violations for which the culture provides no explicit label'.[38] The only commonality uniting such labelling is the use of the concept of mental illness itself. It is the way in which it is employed by members of society and the circumstances in which members resort to its use that should be examined.

Scheff has been accused of saying that there is no such thing as mental illness.[39] He does, in fact, list four types or sources of primary deviance. These are: organic such as genetic, biochemical or physiological conditions; psychological, such as a psychoanalytic interpretation; external stress, such as drugs, combat psychosis and deprivation of sensory stimulation; and volitional acts of innovation or rebellion, such as Dadaism. The concern of the labelling perspective is to focus upon the societal reaction to these acts of residual rule-breaking rather than on the acts themselves. Particular societal attributes are not significant because they cause an individual to commit a deviant act, but because they facilitate or impede that individual's ability to avoid the imposition of a deviant label.

The social contingencies which Scheff identifies as influencing the likelihood of residual rule-breaking being labelled deviant also determine the severity of the societal reaction. These social contingencies are: the degree, amount and visibility of the residual rule-breaking; the power of the residual rule-breaker and the social distance between him and the agents of social control; the tolerance of the community; and the availibility of non-deviant roles. The theoretical perspective in the present study essentially seeks to expand this interpretation. It is proposed to examine the activities of each labelling group in turn with particular attention to the available alternative interpretations of deviance apart from that of being mentally ill. These alternative definitions are likely to be those that best resonate with professional ideologies and best solve the practical problems arising. Rather than label being mentally ill, the police may criminalise behaviour; the family may apportion blame and describe 'wilful' acts; and the social worker may translate conflict into the family dynamics of scapegoating.

Research into the power dimension in the hospitalisation process has produced conflicting interpretations and a level of debate that has resulted in a great deal of heat caused, perhaps, by the frustration of 'talking past each other'.[40] On his side, Scheff has provided evidence of the arbitrary nature of psychiatrists' decision-making in court proceedings.[41] This does not, however, offer direct evidence about the conditions of labelling and the operation of identified social contingencies. One study, which sought to address this problem compared rates of hospitalisation and other 'indicators of psychopathlogy' such as drug arrests, alcoholism, asthma, duodenal ulcer and suicide. The fact that there was no significant correlation was interpreted as evidence of the importance of the societal reaction in determining the level of deviance.[42]

However, in order to examine the process of psychiatric hospitalistion, we must do more than examine large bodies of statistics. Rather, it is necessary to examine the ways in which definitions and categorisations are made, by describing the activities of each labelling group. An ethnomethodological perspective on psychiatric hospitalisation requires an investigation into the interaction, reaction and categorisation that occurs at each stage of the pre-patient phase. Garfinkel argues against a conventional sociology that attempts to transform commmon-sense situations into calculable ones to enable the use of statistical measures. Such an approach, rather than avoiding the distortion of the objective world in a mirror of subjective prejudice, does, in fact, neglect the properties that make events sociological ones.[43] Ethnomethodology seeks to elaborate how members choose among alternative methods of explanation and objectivity, and how they make evident the rational in an organised arrangement. A golden rule of such an approach is that this assessment cannot be made by a rule or standard obtained outside the actual setting.

The meaning of mental illness subsists in the way which the concept is employed. Blum has outlined such an approach: 'mental illness is a sociological phenomena defined in terms of its production . . . in terms of the methods and procedures which members employ to make the phenomenon describable'.[44] These methods and procedures are investigated in terms of the practical reasoning that actors engage in on the basis of their stocks of knowledge, their assemblage of background assumptions and norms which have been conceptualised as their 'sense of social structure'.[45] This involves the study of everyday activities which helps to understand how people make sense of their reality.[46] From this investigation, it may turn out that there is a similarity or uniformity to be discovered about the methods by which members go about such categorising.

The naturalistic approach to deviancy advocates the study of deviants in their natural habitats, but there are clearly difficulties in the present research, unless study is confined to the hospital ward. However, the present concern is the process within home, family and community by which behaviour is reinterpreted as evidence of mental illness and as requiring hospitalisation. This may well be a gradual process, the starting point of which cannot be clearly defined, as has been suggested in the process of becoming delinquent.[47] Such data has to be collected retrospectively because it is clearly not possible for the researcher to sit in on the handling of problems of living in the eventuality that they may be interpreted as evidence of mental illness.[48]

We are, therefore, dependent upon the accounts of patients, relatives, police, social workers and psychiatrists for explanations as to how behaviour comes to be labelled as mentally ill. Such accounts may be analysed in terms of the common-sense precepts that the actor employs in order to appear rational, honest, sensible and decent, as well as to win some interactional advantage. Although the more hard-line ethnomethodologists would deny it, it is surely legitimate to analyse such accounts as demonstrations of actors' beliefs, motives and procedures in the circumstances as described by the actor.[49] From this point of view, there is no substantive difference between accounts of irrational behaviour and rationally motivated action. Both give opportunities to discover the underlying beliefs which govern the ways in which actors choose to describe instances of their activity. It should then be possible to construct propositions to describe the strategies which actors follow in formulating beliefs and undertaking actions in such conditions. An example of such an approach in the interactionist mould is Lemert's description of "becoming paranoid" in terms of an escalating process of exclusion.[50]

This research aims to investigate the ways in which people come to choose, from various methods of understanding, a mental illness interpretation to explain and make rational behaviour and events. An important issue is how this affects the courses of action available to them and the repercussions upon their relationships. The next chapter presents the framework for examining the activities of successive labelling groups on the route to psychiatric hospital.

Notes

1. Kallman, F. (1973) 'The Genetic Theory of Schizophrenia: An analysis of 691 Schizophrenic Twin Index Families, *American Journal of Psychiatry*, 103, 1946. Kallman found that in 86% of his cases where one identical twin was diagnosed as schizophrenic, the other twin was also diagnosed as such. However, there was no effort to control for environment and, in fact, there were only two cases of monozygotic twins reared apart being diagnosed schizophrenic in forty years, which could have been accounted for by chance. As discussed in Coulter, J. *Aspects of Insanity*, London.
2. Ibid. The author quotes the example of researchers seizing on biochemical abnormalities to explain schizophrenia which were in fact due to the effects of hospital diet over a long period of hospitalisation.
3. Goldberg, E. and Morrison, S. (1963) 'Schizophrenia and Social Class', *British Journal of Psychiatry*, 109, pp. 785-802.
4. Dunham, H. (1965) *Community and Schizophrenia: An Epidemiological Analysis*, Detroit.
5. Storle, L., Langner, T., Michael, S. and Opler, M. (1961) *Mental Health in the Metropolis*, New York.
6. Woolf, S. (1973) *Children under Stress*, London.
7. Gay, M. (1967) *Children in Residential Care*, Unpublished prize essay as quoted in Wolf, S. (1973). Three-quarters of the children in a large children's home came from Social Classes IV and V.
8. Department of Health and Social Services (1981) *Hospital Statistics.*
9. Brown, G. and Harris, T. (1978) *Social Origins of Depression*, London.
10. Dohrenwend, B. and Dohrenwend, B. (1969) *Social Status and Psychological Disorder*, New York.
11. Strauss, J. (1979) 'Social and Cultural Influences on Psychopathology ', *Annual Psychological Review*, 30, pp. 397-415.
12. Durkheim, E. (1952) *The Rules of Sociological Method*, New York.
13. Brown, G. and Harris, T. (1978) op. cit. The authors found that working class women were three times more likely to experience a severe household event concerning finance, the home, husband and child, and nearly twice as likely to experience a health difficulty than middle class women.

14. Black, Morris, Smith and Townshend (1983) *Inequalities in Health: The Black Report*, London. The report found that in the first year of life, three times as many babies of Class V parents die as of Class I, and that the rate of chronic sickness was twice as high among unskilled manual workers as the professional classes.
15. Myers, J. and Roberts, B. (1959) *Family and Class Dynamics in Mental Illness*, New York.
16. Hollingshead, A. and Redlich, F. (1958) *Social Class and Mental Ilness*, New York.
17. Gove, W. an Howell, P. (1974) 'Individual Resources and Mental Hospitalisation: A Comparison and Evaluation of the Societal Reaction and Psychiatric Perspectives'. *American Sociological Review*, 39, pp. 86-100.
18. Rushing, W. (1971) 'Individual Resources, Societal Reaction and Hospital Commitment', *American Journal of Sociology*, 77, pp. 511-26. The author argues that the fact that the ratio of involuntary to voluntary hospitalisation increases with lower socio-economic status and being unmarried, is evidence of their lack of power.
19. Hammer, M. (1963) 'The Influence of Small Networks in Mental Hospital Admissions', *Human Organisation*, 22, pp. 243-51.
20. Cohen, S. and Taylor, L. (1973) *Escape Attempts. The Theory and Practice of Resistance to Everyday Life*, London. This approach draws heavily on the author's conceptualisation.
21. Box, S. (1971) *Deviance, Reality and Society*, London, p. 56 ....'Political leaders need to demonstrate their moral and physical superiority by revealing what happens to men who refuse to get into line. So not only do the authorities...incarcerate people who behave in 'odd' ways and call them 'mentally ill', but they need to do so in such a manner that subjects will learn what is officially not tolerated'.
22. Figuera-McDonagh, J. (1978) 'Mental Health among Unemployed Detroiters', *Social Services Review*, Sept. 1978, pp. 383-99. The author found that those unemployed who could get adequate help for daily needs from their primary supports were less psychologically depressed.
23. Strole, L. et al (1961) op. cit.
24. Faris, R. and Dunham, H. (1967) *Mental Disorders in Urban Areas*, Second edition, Chicago.
25. Ibid.
26. Leighton, A. and Leighton, D. (1959) *My Name is Legion*, New York.
27. Blum, A. and McHugh, P. (1971) 'The Social Ascription of Motives', *American Sociological Review*, 36, pp. 98-109, in Atkinson, M. (1982) *Discovering Suicide. Studies in the Social Organisation of Sudden Death*, London, p. 171.
28. Merton, R. (1957) *Social Theory and Social Structure*, New York.
29. Kitsusue, J. and Cicourel, A. (1963) 'A Note on the Uses of Offical Statistics', *Social Problems*, 11, pp. 131-39.

30. Cooper, J. (1970) 'The Use of a Procedure for Standardising Psychiatric Diagnosis', p. 109-31 in *Psychiatric Edipemioloy* edited by Hare and Wing (1970), p. 31. London. The collection of official statistics has a low priority in the hospital in my study; consultants have to be reminded to complete details of diagnosis. These are translated into W.H.O. disease number classification by their medical secretaries. This procedure involves some guesswork. A general diagnosis of depression, for instance, means that a secretary has to choose between one of at least twenty forms of depression from the Glossary of mental disorders.
31. Dohrenwend, B. and Dohrenwend, B. (1970) 'Social and Cultural Influences on Pathology', *Annual Review of Psychology*. 25, pp. 417-52. In a review of 44 studies, the authors found a range of reported prevalence from 1.1 to 69%.
32. Prevalance Surveys (rates per 1,000)

TYPE	AUTHOR	PLACE	DATE	PREV
Low incidence	Hollingshead & Redlich	New Haven Connecticut	1950	8
Medium incidence	Mayer & Gross	Scotland	1948	91
High incidence	Leighton	Stirling Co Nova Scotia	1956	370
High incidence	Rennie et al	Manhatten	1957	750

Hollingshead and Redlich (1958) defined mental illness as those in contact with a psychiatrist as an inpatient or outpatient, public or private. Mayer and Gross (1948) collected information from mental hospitals, school records, general practitioners and public health records. Leighton and Leighton (1959) carried out structured interviews with a sample of the general population to elicit 'hidden symptomatology'. Strole et al (1961) used a similar method of direct interviews.
33. Taylor, L. and Chave, S. (1964) *Mental Health and the Environment*, London.
34. Strole, L. (1961) op. cit.
35. Bastide, R. (1972) *The Sociology of Mental Disorder*. The author has described a two way process; 'the doctor, through the mass media etc., tends to enlarge the field of mental illness by making the public more aware of disturbances that are minor and have until then been attributed to 'oddness or eccentricity'. On the other hand, he accepts the lay definition of mental illness, and his work is limited to refining this definition by introducing categories of 'insanity'. But these categories never extend beyond the boundaries of insanity as defined by public opinion'.
36. Scheff, T. (1966) *Being Mentally Ill*, London.
37. Ibid, p. 33-4.

38. Gove, W. (1970) 'Who is Hospitalised: A Critical Review of some Sociological Studies of Mental Illness', *Journal of Health and Social Behaviour*, 11, pp. 294-303. The author's criticism is that 'primary deviance is attributed to inconsistencies in the social structure, to hedonistic variables, or to ignorance, while psychological characteristics such as personality or psychiatric disorders are ignored'.
39. Gibbs, J. (1981) *The Sociology of Defiance and Social Control*, pp. 483-501 in Social Pathology edited by Rosenburg, M. and Turner, R., New York.
40. Scheff, T. (1964) 'The Societal Reaction to Deviance: Ascriptive Elements in the Screening of Mental Patients in a Mid-western State', *Social Problems*, 11, pp. 3-16.
41. Gibbs, J. (1962) 'Rates of Mental Hospitalisation: A Study of Soietal Reaction to deviant Behaviour', *American Sociologial Review*, 27, pp. 782-92.
42. Garfinkel, H. (1967) *Studies in Ethnomethodology*, New Jersey.
43. Blum, A. (1970) 'The Sociology of Mental Illness' in *Deviance and Respectability* edited by Douglas, J., New York.
44. Cicourel, A. (1968) *The Social Organisation of Juvenile Justice*, New York.
45. Garfinkel, H. (1967) op. cit. The author states: 'Their study (of everyday activities) is directed to the task of learning how members' actual everyday activities consist of methods to make practical actions, practical circumstances, common-sense knowledge of social structures and practical sociological reasoning analyseable, and of discovering the formal properties of common-place, practical common-sense actions from within'.
46. Matza, D. (1964) *Delinquency and Drift*, p. 88. New York. To quote: 'The delinquent process is itself normally a process of gradual development...the first stage may be accidental or unpredictable from the point of view of any theoretical frame of reference, and deflection from the deviant path may be similarly accidental or unpredictable'.
47. There is a strong body of research of this type: e.g. Clausen, J. and Yarrow, M. (1955) 'Mental Illness and the Family', *Journal of Social Issues*, 11, part 1.
48. Wallis, R. and Bruce, S. (1983) 'Accounting for Action: Defending the Commonsense Heresy', *Sociology*, 17, pp. 97-110.
49. Lemert, E. 'Paranoia and the Dynamics of Social Exclusion'.

3 Pathways to hospital

This brief chapter is concerned with providing a structural framework for the description of the activities of successive labellers in the defining of mental illness. The preceding theoretical discussion has outlined the difficulties of a positivist interpretation of the data and has proposed as an alternative an ethnomethodological approach developed out of the labelling perspective. The process of psychiatric hospitalisation is a complicated one which is not easily broken down into component parts. It is a process that has been described as both 'devious and often arbitrary'[1] and characterised as almost fortuitous.[2] Nevertheless, it is important to try and formulate some kind of model which will include all the major factors, and in conclusion an appropiate model will be proposed.

At this stage, the model put forward by Goldberg and Huxley[3] is a useful introduction. It conceptualises the process of psychiatric hospitalisation in terms of five levels and four filters. This model offers a practical solution to the difficulties of structuring such a diffuse and intangible process although it does contain certain inaccuracies and simplifications. It is offered in an adapted form for the present purpose.

Diagram 3.1: Routes to Hospital

	Place and Decision-Maker	Action and Variables
Level 1	Community	Behaviour
Filter 1	Self Relatives Friends and Neighbours Police and Social Services	Attitude to treatment
Level 2	Primary Health Care Setting	Referral
Filter 2	General Practitioner	Attitude and Appraisal by G.P.
Level 3	General Practice	Identified as a case by GP
Filter 3	General Practitioner	Decision to refer to Psychiatric Services
Level 4	Psychiatric Out-Patients Clinic Casualty Departments Other Hospitals	Appraisal & decision to refer for Admission
Filter 4	Psychiatrist	Decision to Admit
	Hospital Doctor	Depending on nosomical contingencies
Level 5	Psychiatric Hospital	Admission

Changes have been made to the original model in order to accommodate the number of referral agents involved in the hospitalisation process. Goldberg and Huxley were concerned primarily with general practice and the role of the G.P., and their presentation gives the impression of a logical and orderly progress through a series of stages and filters. The pre-patient reports to his G.P. who identifies him as a psychiatric case and refers him to the out-patient clinic where the psychiatrist arranges admission if required. However, the results of the present study show that the majority of patients do not pass through all these filters and, more frequently, move directly from Level Three to Level Five, and in extreme cases from Level One to Level Five.

The model is also limited by its failure to consider the alternative outcomes available at each level. The selection process operates to 'filter out' those who do not fulfill the psychiatric criteria as perceived by the labeller. The extent to which such 'filtering- out' occurs is partly determined by the alternative definitions of deviance available and the ideologies and practicalities facing each labelling group. The process of definition and redefinition of behaviour that occurs will be described in the following chapters.

Definition of referral agent in the present study utilises the distinction made by Goffman between complainant and mediator.[4] The complainant is defined as the first person to take effective action aimed at getting someone into hospital and is viewed as referral agent. On the other hand, the mediator is simply the person who facilitates admission and is in most cases a general practitioner. Other studies have tended to group G.P.s as a separate referral group,[5] but this division obscures the activities of other groups. There now follows a breakdown of the patient sample according to referral agent.

Table 3.1: The Patient Sample according to Referral Agent

Referral Agent	Number		Per cent
Self	25		17
Relatives	46		31
Informal Agencies	15		10
(Neighbour/friend)		(10)	
(A.A./Samaritans/Clergy)		(5)	
Formal Agencies	27		18
(Police)		(15)	
(Social Services)		(12)	
Medical Agencies (Other hospitals/ Casualty Units)	9		6
Psychiatric Agencies	27		18
(Out Patient Clinic)		(13)	
(Domiciliary Visits)		(7)	
(Day Hospital/ General Hospital/ Psychiatric Unit)		(7)	

Relatives appear to play the major part in initiating movement towards admission to hospital, followed by formal agencies in which social services play a not insignificant part. The role of formal agencies is reinforced by the fact that nearly one fifth of admissions are from within the psychiatric services. The activities of each of these labelling groups is discussed in detail in the succeeding chapters. Their relative importance in comparison with the findings of other research is now briefly sketched.

Medical sociologists have extensively investigated illness behaviour with respect to physical illness[6] but have largely ignored mental illness. Indeed, the main work in this field remains the pioneering study undertaken by the National Institute of Mental Health in Washington in 1955.[7] The authors, John Clausen and Marion Yarrow, first coined the phrase 'Pathways to Hospital' and were specifically concerned with describing the decision-making leading to hospitalisation, the help-seeking efforts of those involved and the resulting impact of hospitalisation on wife and family. More recent studies, however, have largely ignored how people became patients and concentrated on analysing social characteristics of patient samples.

One example is a study of admissions in a North London Borough,[8] but comparison of results is difficult because of the use of the category of G.P. as a separate referral agent. The proportion of patients being processed through out-patient clinic was somewhat higher than that found in the present study: 27.5 per cent as compared to 18 per cent. Entry into psychiatric hospital via other hospital doctors was also twice as high in North London. The authors of a study of attempted suicide in Northern Ireland report that over 80 per cent of such cases coming through the Casualty Unit were referred for psychiatric assessment, some 20 per cent subsequently became psychiatric inpatients, and a further 50 per cent psychiatric out-patients.[9] With nearly three-quarters of the sample having become in or out-patients, overdosing was an effective way of achieving psychiatric contact. Both studies confirm that the proposed model of selective filtering outlined by Goldberg and Huxley only applies in a minority of cases.

It is important to emphasise the ability of the individual himself to influence outcome, a factor which tends to be glossed over in a purely epidemiological approach. American research has, more often, recognised the significance of the individual. For instance, Hollingshead and Redlich investigated the relation between social class and path to hospital and found that lower class patients were more often involved in admission via the police and higher class patients more often referred themselves or were referred by their families.[10]

A final aspect of the admission process to be considered is that of type of admission. Mental Health legislation specifically provides for the compulsory or 'formal' admission of patients to hospital against their will. General Practitioners are invested with the legal powers to refer patients for compulsory admission. Hospital doctors may overturn the G.P.'s decision and admit voluntarily a person referred for compulsory admission, but they also have the authority to detain a voluntary patient..

Table 3.2: Patient Sample according to Type of Admission

Type of Admission	Number	Per Cent
Voluntary	111	74
Compulsory	29	20
Compulsory admissions regraded to voluntary on admission	6	4
Voluntary admissions made compulsory within first week of admission	3	2

A study of compulsory admissions in the London area found that over half of such admissions did not meet the criteria laid down in the Act.[11] The author concluded that there was evidence of the rules being misused albeit from altruistic motives, some doctors feeling that theirs was a higher duty to the welfare of the patient. However, concentration only on the figure of compulsory admissions draws attention away from the element of compulsion that may have been used in 'voluntary' admissions by the use of such strategies as 'if you don't come into hospital voluntarily, I'll sign you in'. The use of compulsion suggests that people resist stigmatising labels and have to be compelled to adopt them. In the present study, the fact that in six cases the admitting doctor was able to admit a detained patient voluntarily suggests that label resistance had evaporated by the time hospital was reached. On the other hand, the fact that 2 per cent of voluntary admissions were subsequently made compulsory shows that occassionally resistance increases. These issues will be discussed further in the section on the formal agencies. Finally, the figure for compulsory admissions was considerably higher at 20 per cent than the 12% reported in England.[12]

Patient Career

To complete the picture, the hospital characteristics of the patient sample are described in terms of diagnosis and length of admission. Previous research has found that rehospitalisation is related to duration and number of previous admissions, the longer and more frequent a person has been in hospital, the more likely he is to return.[13] Both these aspects of patient career are also described.

Table 3.3: Patient Sample and Number of Previous Admissions

Admissions	Number	Per cent
None	43	29
1-2	44	33
3-4	31	21
5-9	14	9
over 10	17	11

Table 3.4: Patient Sample and Length of Previous Hospitalisation

Total Time in Hospital	Number	Per cent
None	44	29
under 1 month	22	15
1-3 months	21	14
3-6 months	31	21
under 1 year	16	11
1-2 years	10	7
over 2 years	4	3

The two tables present a picture of two distinctive groups of patients. On the one hand, between a quarter and a third of those coming into hospital have had no previous experience of psychiatric hospitalisation although upwards of a quarter had been previous patients in other psychiatric hospitals. This compares with a figure for first admissions of 40 per cent in North London.[14] Studies in Dublin have shown a high rate of first admissions when compared internationally.[15] On the other hand, there was a clearly identifiable group of 'revolving-door' or 'disguised long-stay' patients who made up a tenth of the sample. An American study found that 65 per cent of patients are likely to be readmitted within five years and described this feature as 'intermittent patienthood.[16]

Table 3.5: Patient Sample and Length of Stay in Hospital

Time	Number	Per cent
1 week and under	18	12
1-2 weeks	23	15
2-3 weeks	23	16
3-4 weeks	19	13
4-9 weeks	33	22
10 weeks to 6 months	16	10
over 6 months	7	5
over 2 years	10	7

The picture is one of short admission with a quarter of the sample being in hospital less than two weeks. On the other hand, 21 per cent of patients had a total period in hospital of more than six months and 20 per cent of patients had more than five admissions to hospital. Although these two groups are not necessarily the same this is another indication of short and frequent admission. It is important to remember that these figures are from an acute admission ward and do not take into consideration the average length of stay of the total hospital population. Overall, it has been found in the Republic of Ireland that some 70 per cent of the hospital population has been in hospital over twenty years.[17] American research has emphasised the connection between lower social class and long-term hospitalisation; if discharged the lower class patient is more likely to be isolated from formal and informal groups in the community.[18]

Table 3.6: Patient Sample according to Diagnosis

Diagnosis	Number	Per cent
Functional Psychoses (chiefly schizophrenia)	31	21
Affective psychoses (depression and mania)	34	23
Neuroses	16	10
Personality Disorder	22	15
Alcohol/drug abuse	35	23
Other	3	2

Two groups of conditions predominate: major organic illnesses and psychotic disorders, which are later described as 'genuine' mental illness, account for nearly half of admissions: Personality disorders and addictive states, which are later described as 'undesirable' admissions and form the remainder of 40 per cent. The neuroses, which make up a tenth of the sample, fill a middle position in terms of acceptability to psychiatrists between the 'genuine' mental illnesses and the 'undesirable' personality disorders. There is often a conflict of interest between the demands of patients and the demands of professional groups. How this is negotiated is a major preoccupation of this study.

The group consisting of personality disorders and problems of addiction is reported as making up an increasing proportion of hospital admissions in the post-war period.[19] The recent study in North London found a smaller proportion of patients diagnosed 'personality disorder', 9 per cent of admissions, and a corresponding increase in the figure for those diagnosed as suffering from affective disorders; 42 per cent of admissions.[20] Comparison between hospitals must, however, be treated with care because of differences in the diagnostic habits of medical personnel.

The patient sample is divided between those who are experiencing their first contact with psychiatric hospital, which is likely to be relatively short and not repeated, and those who experience frequent admissions of varying duration. It is likely that length of hospitalisation is related to diagnosis.

Summary

This chapter has been concerned with providing a structural framework for the portrayal of the dynamics of the social process of psychiatric hospitalisation. The following chapters will continue the theme of describing the activities of the labelling groups of self, family, neighbours and other informal groups. The activities of the main gatekeeper, the general practitioner, will then be highlighted followed by an investigation of the operation of the formal agencies of police, social workers and finally psychiatrists themselves.

Notes

1. Kessel, N. (1963) 'Who Ought to see a Psychiatrist', *Lancet*, 18.5.1963, pp. 1092-5.
2. Clausen, J. and Yarrow, M. (1955) 'Paths to the Mental Hospital', *Journal of Social Issues*, 11, pp. 25-32.
3. Goldberg, D. and Huxley, P. (1980) *Mental Illness in the Community*. London.
4. Goffman, E. (1961) *Asylums*, New York.
5. Mezey, A. and Evans, E. (1971) 'Psychiatric in-Patients and Out-patients in a London Borough', *British Journal of Psychiatry*, pp. 609-16.
6. Tuckett, D. (1976) *Introduction to Medical Sociology*, London.
7. Clausen, J. and Yarrow, M. (1955) 'Impact of Mental Illness on the Family', *Journal of Social Issues*, 11, part No. 4.
8. Mezey, A. and Evans, E. (1971) op. cit.
9. Robinson, K. and Savage, M. (1985) 'Aspects of Attempted Suicide in Northern Ireland', D.H.S.S. *Occasional Papers*, No. 30.
10. Hollingshead, A. and Redlich, F. (1958) *Social Class and Mental Illness*, Chapt. 6. New York.
11. Bean, P. (1980) *Compulsory Admissions to Mental Hospitals*, London.
12. Department of Health and Social Services (1979) *Psychiatric Hospital Statistics*.
13. Rosehblatt, A. and Meyer, J. (1974) 'The Recidivism of Mental Patients: a Review of Past Studies', *American Journal of Orthopsychiatry*, 44, pp. 697-706.
14. Mezey, A. and Evans, E. (1971) op. cit.
15. Walsh, D. (1969) 'Mental Illness in Dublin - First Admissions', *British Journal of Psychiatry*, 115, pp. 449-56.
16. Friedman, I., Mering, O. and Hinko, E. (1966) 'Intermittent Patienthood', *Archive General Psychiatry*, 14, pp. 386-392.
17. O'Hare, A. and Walsh, D. (1971) *Irish Psychiatric Census*.
18. Myers, J. and Bean, L. (1968) *A Decade Later: A Follow-up of Social Class and Mental Illness*, New York.
19. Kramer, M. (1955) 'A Historical Study of the Dispositions of First Admissions to a State Mental Hospital', *Public Health Monogram*, No. 32.
20. Mezey, A. and Evans, E. (1971) op. cit.

4 The patient

In a sense, we begin at the end by first describing the position of the central character - the patient - and his attempts to understand and deal with his predicament. The term 'patient' implies a passive endurance which neglects the potential of the individual to determine and influence what is happening to him. An alternative description may be the 'perpetrator' which conveys a sense of the ownership of acts committed. In the first half of the chapter, I propose to examine the particular characteristics of the group of perpetrators who actively sought their own admission. The second half is concerned with an investigation of the strategies used by psychiatric patients to deal with their stigmatised and negative status.

Self-labelling

Labelling theorists have tended to preclude the possibility of self-labelling occuring before social labelling. The Scheffian position views the role of the psychiatric patient as a negative and stigmatised status which the individual has to be persuaded to perform, according to a stereotyped imagery learnt in childhood, by a system of rewards and punishments. The fact that individuals are persuaded to enter such a negative role is explained by their highly suggestible and vulnerable state at the time of labelling when they see no alternative to such labelling.[1] Scheff draws upon social-psychological research which has found that the public hold to an uncompromisingly negative picture of the mentally ill.[2] More recent research shows some evidence of public discrimination between mental illness labels [3], and an examination of the causal models utilised by the public to explain mental illness has shown that the public follow an eclectic approach.[4]

Studies of the portrayal of the mentally ill in the mass media have found that a negative stereotype predominates.[5] Although the developmental explanation of human behaviour, as presented in the psychoanalytical model, has become of enormous importance in America, this 'psychologism'[6] has not replaced more moralistic explanations. The Hollywood psychodrama, typified by Alfred Hitchcock's film 'Psycho', remains a potent force shaping public attitudes but such stereotypes have become mixed with 'psychologism' and the effects of mental health education programmes. There is some evidence that, whilst there exists some broad congruence between public knowledge and psychiatric symptomatology, this agreement tends to be over one particular category of mental illness, namely schizophrenia.[7] Thomas Scheff in his elaboration of a labelling theory of mental illness is also primarily concerned with schizophrenia and recurring episodes of mental disorder.[8]

Research into public attitudes towards defining mentally ill behaviour conveys an impression of a public which prefers to have its labelling done for it, and, in corollary, the public is only sure that someone is mentally ill when he has been placed in a psychiatric hospital.[9] A pioneering attempt to broaden public attitudes towards mental illness through an education programme foundered on the proposition that normal and abnormal behaviour were not distinct but fell within a single continuum.[10] The degree of hostility expressed against such a notion suggests that clear cut-off points between abnormal and normal behaviour had a functional purpose. Denial allows society to maintain an appearance of integrity until deviation cannot be ignored, when the deviant is removed and isolated.[13] The act of labelling and removal also provides an opportunity to reaffirm social norms and to highlight the boundary between normal and abnormal behaviour.

Labelling theory has been criticised for 'conveying a process which is unilateral, which leaves no place for human choice, and which results in a systematic inattention to the rule-breaker's definition of, and reactions to, the labelling process'.[12] However, any discussion of self-motivation to enter the mentally ill role needs to concentrate on the possible advantages of the sick role which may outweigh the disadvantages of an associated negative and stigmatised status. Talcott Parsons conceptualised the sick role as a partly legitimised status with a system of rights and obligations.[13] The advantages for the individual of being sick are exemption from normal social responsibilities, exemption from responsibility for the illness, and legitimation of 'the need to be taken care of'. Such legitimised benefits are rare. Entry to the sick role is circumscribed and only validated by a doctor. There are also certain obligations on the individual in the sick role 'to want to get well' and to seek technical help.

Particular and special importance is attached to these obligations in the field of mental illness where the patient's attitude to his predicament is, of itself, a significant variable in defining illness. The absence of 'insight' may, in fact, be a crucial determinant of illness. There is a second important difference in the sick role for the mentally ill as opposed to the physically ill and that is the way in which the mentally ill role may become a predominant and permanent status for the individual, what Scheff describes as a master status, rather than a temporary and partially legitimised status as described by Parsons.[14]

The positive and negative aspects of the sick role for the mentally ill are clearly of crucial importance in determining the individual's motivation to enter such a role. Whilst the suspension of responsibilities and the opportunity for dependence may be considerable incentives, they must be weighed against the likelihood of being stuck with a negative and stigmatised status. Recent work on self-labelling emphasises the importance of a previously held negative self-conceptualisation as increasing the likelihood of self-labelling.[15]

Through an intrapsychic process the actor reasons with himself about the way in which he is behaving. This process of self-interaction[16] involves the actor in a reflexive process by which he reasons and compares himself to an imagined or known ideal figure. If his evaluation is negative, then, new negative evaluations are more likely to be incorporated and self-labelling is more likely to occur. If it is positive, the likelihood of transformative labelling taking place depends on the influence of significant others. Rotenburg suggests that such labelling is only likely to occur when the labeller is a primary other to the labelee (primary persons being those whose valuative reactions are incorporated into the actor's self-identity).[17] Rotenburg's view would suggest that the likelihood of self-labelling occurring following labelling by official social agents is reduced because such agents are secondary others to the labelee. In the case of Alcoholics Anonymous, the deliberate use of stigmatised labels to reduce deviance depends on the importance of the labeleee being a voluntary participant and the labeller being a member of the labelled category.[18]

The advantages of the sick role, relationship with labeller,and prior self-conceptualisation have all been identified as significant factors in encouraging acceptance of label. Self-labelling is a vivid part of hospital life. At the time of writing, one young man only discharged an hour previously and removed from the hospital by the police, jumped in through a window of the ward in his efforts to be readmitted. This is a rather startling example of self-labelling but statistical evidence from the study sample indicated that some 17 per cent of admissions were initiated by the perpetrator and hence could be seen as self-labelling.

Comparative statistics are difficult to find because of the lack of research in this area and unclear definitions of agent of hospitalisation. Two British surveys in Scotland[19] and London[20] group self-referrers with others in a residual category which does not distinguish between complainant and mediator. American research in this field is facilitated by the fact that self-referral directly to hospital is common. For example, a retrospective study in Washington found that some 11 per cent of admissions were at the patient's initiative.[21] On the West Coast of America research indicates that people presenting themselves for admission have previously been in hospital and fall into the category of 'revolving-door patients'.[22] This group would conform to the Scheffian view which concentrates attention on 'careers of chronic deviance'. A distinction may usefully be drawn between the Scheffian group of 'revolving door' patients and an alternative group of self-labellers who may be described as 'outsiders' because they have difficulty persuading others of their right to the sick role.

Before examining these two groups in detail, it is important to identify a number of broad influences on self-labelling. In the first place, Parsons has argued that an individual's motivation to enter the sick role is related to his life stage.[23] The sick role is similar to the childhood role encouraging a state of dependency which may be particularly appealing. The sick role represents the major opportunity in our society for the individual to be legitimately absolved from his responsibilities. Its importance has been enhanced by the medicalisation of new areas of human activity[24] and by the institutionalisation of the right to free medical care and treatment in most Western countries. In Scheffian terms, the sick role has become one of the major alternative forms of deviance available to individuals and one that is, moreover, semi-legitimating. The extent to which individuals will seek to enter the sick role will also be influenced by social variables such as social class[25] and the structure of community networks.[26]

Instances of self-labelling are complex and involve interactional processes which are difficult to unravel. Consider an individual coming into hospital for the first time and the way his voluntary participation interplays with family pressure to ensure entry to hospital.[27]

> "I imagined that I had all sorts of things wrong with me, like cancer.I had my own doctor tormented, he gave me tablets but they were no good. All these worries kept coming up - things weren't right at home and I couldn't go to work. I wanted a check-up and the doctor ordered me in here; I was that much worked up that I wouldn't stay and walked home. They talked to me again and I came back a third time.I was then told that my wife had signed a form so that the hospital could stop me leaving. I could see no way out of it; I couldn't sit or do anything; I felt just like ending it all. I imagine that I've had some sort of nervous breakdown - my nerves seemed to get the better of me".

This case demonstrates the way in which complaints are viewed by the patient in terms of physical illness but are reinterpreted by his doctor as psychiatric symptomatology. This reinterpretation is resisted by the patient but the efforts of his wife, which represents the evaluative judgement of a primary other, succeed in persuading him to return to hospital. Scheff would argue that the individual is particularly vulnerable at the time of labelling, being at the centre of a crisis in which he is highly suggestible. The efforts of relatives, and the individual's desperate need for help culminate in the use of compulsory powers to achieve hospitalisation. The individual is left with no alternative and, by the time of the interview at the end of his treatment, he too has accepted a psychiatric definition of his behaviour.

The above case illustrates the interplay of various factors in the process of hospitalisation. The prepatient's motivation to enter hospital is one of these factors. In the breakdown of cases where self-labelling is the dominating factor, two distinctive features are apparent. Instances of self-labellling commonly occur either where the individual has previously achieved legitimised psychiatric status and is seeking his own return to hospital, or where the efforts of the individual to achieve hospitalisation are discouraged and even resisted by hospital staff. The characteristics of these two groups are now examined.

The Revolving Door Patient

It is not surprising that number of previous admissions is an important predictor of the likelihood of rehospitalisation,[28] nor is it surprising that as individuals stay in hospital they increasingly adopt the prevailing psychiatric ideology, and it has been shown that those who are most positive are more likely to be readmitted quicker at a later date.[29] These features are illustrated in the following case

> Mr 'F' had been in hospital twenty times although never for more than a few weeks at a time. He was diagnosed as suffering from chronic schizophrenia. On this occasion, after his landlord had threatened him with eviction he presented himself to his Doctor and asked to be admitted to hospital as he was feeling depressed about the threat of eviction. He made his own way to the hospital with an introductory letter from his G.P. Once admitted in hospital, he explained that 'a wee stay would help me as things have got on top of me and I think too much'. He saw the supervision in hospital as helping to "steady him up" and expected to make a speedy recovery. Mr 'F' was discharged within two weeks.

Mr 'F' has achieved the right of quick and legitimate entry to the patient role which he readily embraces in times of difficulty. Such 'revolving door' patients are characteristically diagnosed schizophrenic and such a label is a prerequisite to easy access to hospital. The process of achieving such a status is demonstrated by another case of a young woman, similarly diagnosed, who was in hospital three times during the survey period. On the first occasion, her social worker facilitated her admission; the second time, she was admitted via casualty; by the third admission, she was accepted on the strength of her own telephone call direct to the ward.

A second factor influencing the likelihood of self-referral is the importance of the individual in his own family and wider networks. His own awareness of his need for outside help may be brought home more readily by his inability to perform important duties. Hammer has suggested that the more important the patient is to his family, the quicker he will come into hospital.[30] In the present group there are two examples of this type. Both involve married men with children, both of whom unemployed, although maintaining some functional importance as father with child-rearing responsibilities.

Revolving door patients possess labels of 'genuine' mental illness which facilitate their ready return to hospital. This is not the case with the second group whose act of self labelling is not, of itself, sufficient to achieve their desired aim of hospital admission.

The Outsiders

Given that 'being sick' is our main source of relief from environmental and interpersonal problems that may seem insurmountable, it is not surprising that some people demand the right of entry to psychiatric hospital. These self-labellers divide into those who present a problem of alcohol abuse and those who directly report overwhelming environmental pressures. Both groups are faced with similar problems in achieving the reinterpretation of their behaviour into medical terms.

The principle objective of the petitioner is to achieve the translation of his behaviour from moral terms to symptoms of illness. This is well illustrated by a husband seeking admission for his drunken wife who argues with staff that 'she's not drunk, she's ill'. It can be seen that the degree to which the petitioner succeeds in achieving a medical translation of his behaviour is influenced by various institutional factors. In the case of alcoholism these include professional pessimism about the efficacy of treatment and a consequent reluctance to admit such long term sufferers.

The return to a more moral viewpoint of alcoholism has, on the one hand, resulted in sufferers engaging other strategies to be admitted, and, on the other hand, staff searching for other motives for their being in hospital. Those seeking admission may act, or threaten to act, in a dramatic way to translate their behaviour into psychiatric terms. Effectively, this has meant acting in a para-suicidal manner:

> Mr 'X' had nineteen previous admissions to hospital for alcoholism. Following his last drinking bout he asked his G.P. to admit him into hospital. When refused, he returned the following day to the surgery threatening to harm himself if he was not admitted. His G.P. acquiesced and arranged admission. When his wife was interviewed she said she believed "he went into hospital to escape her financial control" and to save for his next drinking spree. Her opinion of his motivation encouraged the hospital, after a few days, to quickly discharge him.

Sufferers are expected to want to get well and take responsibility for their predicament.[31] In such a climate, the petitioner is likely to go where he anticipates a sympathetic response, in one case returning from England and walking most of the way to the hospital.

The second group of outsiders, those overwhelmed by environmental and interpersonal problems, has a similar problem in negotiating hospital admission and acts in a similar way. Taking an overdose draws attention to the individual's plight, and imitates psychiatric behaviour. The individual is brought into the medical ambit where temporary relief of responsibility for problems may be granted. At one Northern Ireland hospital 70% of those admitted following overdose or self-injury became either psychiatric in-patients or out-patients.[32] Such studies of overdosing behaviour show deteriorating relationships to be the main precipitating factor.[33] Although the effects of unemployment and financial deprivation are not directly apparent, they may well be mediated through relationship problems.[34] All these features are present in the following example which also illustrates one strategy for seeking help.

> This young single mother had been told by her boyfriend that he wanted to end their relationship and she had been in conflict with her own family over him. She was also in debt and in danger of losing her employment. As a result, she had started another job at night. She said that she felt that she 'just couldn't cope anymore, that she didn't want to know anybody and that she didn't care what was going to happen to her". She described 'Everything closing in on her' and took some tablets and went to the Health Centre. She then sought out a doctor who previously had been sympathetic to her and he arranged for her to come into hospital directly.

Direct admission from hospital casualty unit following an incident of self-harm circumvents a G.P. who may be regarded as unsympathetic by the petitioner. Psychiatric assessment is routine in most general hospitals in such cases and may well result in a more ready reinterpretation and entry into hospital than would otherwise take place. In one instance, a G.P. was advised by a hospital doctor to arrange psychiatric admission for a woman who had discharged herself before psychiatric referral could be made.

The primary problem for the group of self-labellers is achieving legitimation of their desire to occupy the sick role. I have described this activity in terms of a number of strategies which may invoke opposing organisational strategies. Such institutional responses will be discussed in the following chapters as the activities of each occupational group are examined in turn. Of crucial importance for the petitioner is the possibility of abdication of responsibility for actions and predicament, an absolution, which may operate retrospectively. Previous acts for which the actor has been maligned in terms of making a nuisance, being blamed for or acting out of badness are now redefined as being symptoms of illness which require the sympathy of others. These are high rewards and it is not surprising that the petitioner may go to considerable lengths to achieve them.

Strategies for Psychological Survival

While some may find advantage in being 'sick', they may also find that hospitalisation threatens their own self-esteem. Social-psychological studies of patient attitudes are sparse but two main points seem clear: patients share the negative attitudes of the public towards mental illness; and they tend to deny their mental illness in the same way as the public.

These findings can be broadly summarised as follows: patients evaluate the mentally ill in negative terms;[35] locked ward patients hold a more moralistic approach to mental illness than open ward patients;[36] the discrepancy between staff and patient attitudes declines during hospitalisation, the latter being typically influenced by the former;[37] those patients who express the most favourable attitudes towards treatment are likely to experience the shortest stay;[38] and patients are as eclectic as the general public when it comes to conceptual models of mental illness.[39] These findings have all been confirmed in an Irish context.[40]

> "If you say you're well , the doctor will keep you in hospital. If you say you're ill, you'll get out quicker"

The conundrum facing the psychiatric patient is summed up in this quote from one patient. Admission of illness may lead to early discharge but such an admission will call into question individual personal and psychological self-identity. Therefore, the patient searches for strategies for psychological protection but these strategies may themselves be interpreted as further proof of illness.

Unlike physical medicine where patient attitude to health is less of a factor in symptomatology, the psychiatric patient's attitude to his illness has a particular importance. Psychiatrists use the term 'insight' to convey the extent to which the patient shows his belief and understanding that his past behaviour is caused by mental illness, and the growth of 'insight' is used as one measure of his progress in hospital. The psychiatrist seeks out the patient's attitude to the validity of his thoughts and actions in order to test the patient's relationship to 'concrete reality'. Given that schizophrenia is used as a category to describe people who persistently believe in the reality of their disturbed thoughts, the person labelled schizophrenic is often not in a position to show this awareness. It is in this sense that schizophrenia is a chronic and permanent status and, hence, the conundrum posed in the quotation.

Given the wide variety of behaviour arriving in psychiatric hospital, the psychiatrist's response to cases clearly varies. In one set of circumstances, he may seek to persuade an individual of his illness while in another situation he may deny the illness label. However, whether a person is a willing, reluctant, or unwilling resident in psychiatric hospital he is still faced with the same problems in maintaining his psychological identity and sense of self esteem.

Patient activity has been notably documented by Erving Goffman with his portrayal of an inmate world with its own unique features and individual identity, founded against the prevailing institutional regime.[41] Goffman asserts that 'our status is backed by the solid buildings of the world, while our sense of personal identity resides in the cracks.[42] A similar approach is adopted by Taylor and Cohen in their study of long term prisioners in which they are concerned with 'how life is given meaning, how one passes the time, how friends are made and lost, how one resigns oneself to the environment and how one resists it'.[43] A more recent study of a group of short term female psychiatric patients pointed out a number of ways in which the negative and stigmatising aspects of the psychiatric patient role were resisted.[44] Such an approach emphasises the importance of individual reactions to labelling and recognises the potential for individuals to resist labelling and to escape from deviant roles, and, in certain instances, the ways they may unintentionally induce labelling. This approach counters the more deterministic bias of a pure labelling perspective in order to 'recognise the full humanity of the deviant . . that he be seen as active as well as passive, as subject as well as object, and as producer as well as product'.[45] If we look at the ways in which the patient sample saw their own situation, three broad categories of interpretation are found. This breakdown is outlined in the following table.

Table 4.1: Problem Behaviour for Self

Problem behaviour	Number	Per cent	
Physical ill-health	28	24)	
Adverse change in material circumstances	20	17)	41%
Loneliness/unable to look after self	19	16)	28%
Breakdown in relationships	14	12)	
Feelings of persecution and fear	20	17)	
Feelings of sin, guilt and hopelessness	15	14)	31%

Patients' interpretations of their situations can be linked to strategies adopted to maintain their integrity in hospital. Broadly, the first group of 41% emphasised external problems of physical ill-health and adverse material circumatances to explain their hospital admission. This group are 'label resistors 'who adopt a physical ailment explanation or a social causation explanation. Both views aim to explain predicament in everyday terms and thereby to normalise behaviour. The second group of 28%, offer explanations of loneliness, poor relationships and inability to look after themselves, and may be taking on part of the responsibility for their breakdown. The third group of 31% reported classic psychiatric symptoms of guilt, hopelessness and fears of persecution and may be viewed as potential 'label acceptors', in so far as they have gone along with the medical explanation for their feelings. Each of the main strategies of psychological survival will now be discussed in turn with illustrations from the case material.

i) Label Acceptance

Previous research has indicated a natural history of resistance to institutional definitions. The labelled individual is gradually worn down and overcome in the hospital so that he is eventually forced to take on the psychiatric staff's view of his personal history and behaviour.[46] The revolving-door patient may be viewed in this way. For example, a patient stated:

'I knew I wasn't well when I arrived here in hospital again. I thought these things going on inside my head were real until I got here. You speak to that many people you don't know what to think. For instance, I spoke to my cousin and she said she didn't think I was mentally ill at all, but I believe it when I speak to the doctor, after all he's the psychiatrist.'

The fact of hospitalisation and the authority of the doctor bring about an acceptance of the 'definition of mentally ill'. The role of psychiatric patient gives relief from responsibilities for actions that is not forthcoming outside hospital. This label acceptance occurs through a process of self-interaction in which the individual compares his present behaviour with the way he previously behaved. He also compares it with the behaviour of significant others and takes into account their definitions of his behaviour.

How far acceptance of the definition of being mentally ill represents an invalidation of self depends on the extent to which being a psychiatric patient is a master status. There are a number of ways in which the individual can successfully deal with the attendant stigma and negative status. One of these is by role distance or 'hamming it up', illustrated by one patient who said: 'it's a bit like a club in here - the "over the moon club" except the cocktails aren't served until ten o' clock'.

An alternative strategy which allows the actor to accept a stigmatising label whilst maintaining his overall sense of self-worth is compartmentalisation. What is happening in one area of life which is unsatisfactory and stigmatising can be kept separate from other constituent parts of the individual so that his overall identity is kept intact. This 'double bookkeeping' is commonly observed in hospital. The patient continues to believe his thoughts and actions and denies illness at the same time as accepting hospitalisation and taking medication.

In certain instances, a stigmatising label may be deliberately used in a positive way to produce conventional behaviour by enforcing acceptance of a deviant label. The most clear-cut example is Alcoholics Anonymous where solidarity between labelled alcoholics and the blurring of distinctions between labeller and labellee play a very important part in the AA philosophy. For example, one patient stated ' only another alcoholic understands how you feel: when I get the obsession to drink I turn to my friends in AA and the whole yearning goes'. I will return to the importance of solidarity for the patient group.

ii) Label Resistance

Resistance to the label of mentally ill may take a number of forms. The patient may rely on an interpretation of his behaviour that is less stigmatising; that he is suffering from a physical illness, for example. Alternativly, the individual may seek explanation in causes outside of himself, such as social factors, and thereby achieve the normalisation of behaviour. A third possibility for the patient is outright denial of the label.

As previously cited research has indicated, the public does not regard mental illness as being similar to physical illness. Mental illness calls into question the individual's self-identity in a way that being physically ill does not. Physically ill people can distance themselves from their symptoms which are bodily malfunctions which do not reflect on them or lead to the apportionment of blame. As these advantages are readily available for the physically sick, those labelled mentally ill may well reinterpret their hospitalisation in terms of physical illness in order to enjoy those benefits. For example, asked to explain why they were in hospital, one patient answered: - 'I had a bad chest which affects me and weighs me down I can't get my work done' and another said 'I came into hospital because I am a very sick man - I couldn't sleep at night and I want the doctors to get my sleep right'

The folk terminology of mental illness invokes mechanistic and physical explanations. Patients frequently speak of 'being bad with the nerves' and the term 'nervous breakdown' is in widespread use. Such linguistics link mental and physical illness by picturing nervous disorders as bodily malfunctioning.

The strategy of seeking casual explanation outside oneself is one that is enshrined in the Alcoholics Annonymous message. Bateson has described how AA see alcoholism as 'an existential battle with the bottle, in which the alcoholic must learn that he cannot beat the bottle, but that he must move from a symmetrical to a complementary relationship and submit to it's domination'.[47] The AA message has been incorporated in the medical model of alcoholism as a disease. The bottle is like a virus outside of the person. One patient summarised this view:

> "I was a member of AA for a year and I hadn't taken a drink. Things were going that good that I took a bender. I know now that I cannot drink; plenty of meetings, they're the answer - one every night because that's where I belong. I have a disease and I have to live with it".

One of the main ways of placing cause outside oneself is to blame social factors and such social causation explanations have three components of interest. In the first place, common-sense theorising reflects those sociological explanations of mental illness that emphasise stress and deprivation as causal factors. Secondly, such social explanations place cause outside oneself, which enables the individual to protect his self-worth. Bean reported that patients described their hospitalisation in terms of 'time out' from day-to-day pressures and that they saw their illness as located in 'the sociomoral world of their everyday experience'.[48] Finally, it may be asserted that being overwhelmed by social troubles is understandable and 'could happen to anyone', hence such behaviour is 'normal'. In the present study, two main factors, poverty and loneliness, were emphasised by patients. Here, is a case example:

> "The hopelessness of trying to live on supplementary benefit overwhelmed me. When my son leaves school this year it will be reduced again. At the moment, after deductions for rent and electricity, I'm left with only £28 a week to live on. Before I came

> into hospital, I went to Social Services to ask for help but they told me they could not give me a grant. If I had had someone to talk to, I would have been O.K. but I had nowhere to turn and took an overdose."

There are two processes at work: normalisation and medicalisation. Hospitalisation is caused by very real problems but these problems are integrated into a medical illness account. The following statement by a patient describes this process.

> "I live on my own and it's very, very lonely - I don't bother with anybody and the only outlet is the people I meet when I go for a drink. I can't cope with the outside world on my own and I think that loneliness is a disease in itself. My car was stolen and my other car set on fire. That happening to anyone would make them crack."

Many patients use denial to keep at bay the hurtful conflicts and anxieties, which result from the inferior social status of the mentally ill.[49]. One way in which self esteem can be maintained is to establish a hierarchy of mental illness with themselves placed in the most acceptable category. For instance, one patient said: 'it helps you to see people worse off than yourself'. However, whilst some patients might believe that their relatives had the same positive perception of themselves as they had, others blamed their relatives for their hospitalisation.

Denial brings with it the assertion that one is still in control; the passivity attached to the role of being mentally ill can be rejected. Even when it is impossible to deny their problems, some patients may still insist that these problems result from their own poor decisions and their own ineffective action. For example:

> "After a day or two in hospital this thing just hit me like a nervous breakdown. Before that you wouldn't have said I was a bad case at all. I let myself get into a bad state of nerves, I should have kept battling."

Assertion of control means missing out on relief of responsibility for one's predicament. This burden must remain with the individual and must remain a significant stress, a stress which may be greater than the stress caused by the stigma of accepting the psychiatric patient status.

Expressing Solidarity

Patients may cope with their stigmatised status by developing a solidarity with other patients in hospital. This solidarity may be manifested in what Goffman calls 'the underlife of the institution'[50]. Cigarettes play an important part in the daily interaction between patients and may well represent something with which staff cannot interfere. Patients readily offer help to each other and express sympathy for each others' predicament. Solidarity may also be displayed against the institution: a reluctance to attend programmes; a ridiculing of demands made; a mimicking of staff and so on. At the same time, patients are sensitive towards the power relationship in hospital and some evidence of this was found in my interviewing when patients were generally reluctant to express open criticism of the hospital regime.

The growth of solidarity between patients is a feature of hospitalisation which has been overlooked by Talcott Parsons who argued that the sick role is a less harmful form of deviance for society precisely because it is not likely to lead to 'a solidary sub-culture of similarly oriented deviants'.[51] For Parsons the patient's main bond is to the doctors and other staff rather than to other patients, although he admitted to the possible exception of 'magic-mountain like communities'[52] What he meant by this phrase is not made clear but the psychiatric hospital in which people live together for long periods in lessening degrees of incapacity, does offer the opportunity for solidarity to grow amongst patients. T.B. sanatoria offer similar opportunities; in both settings the patient experiences remissions during which they are well and behave as a healthy person, at the same time as continuing to retain their patient identity and be part of institutional life.[53]

The solidarity within hospital may survive for a time outside with discharged patients visiting each other. This may be because they are isolated by the stigma of mental illness from their pre-hospitalisation social networks. It would seem that speedy and successful reintegration into conventional society depends on a casting-off of the stigmatised identity of psychiatric patient. The extent to which this reintegration can happen is partly determined by the attitudes of those who make up the individual's social network. Interestingly, doctors routinely discourage patients from maintaining friendships made in hospital, perhaps to encourage integration or to tie the patient into the doctor/patient relationship. However, self help groups like AA are now reasonably widespread, and the solidarity of youth may survive the separation of discharge.

Attempts to build on such solidarity to positively transform the psychiatric patient identity in a political sense have been made by the pressure group MIND which has been significantly successful in the promotion of the rights of patients. However, the main activists were lobbyists with a concern for civil liberties, although there are increasingly actively involved ex-patients who proclaim their hospitalisation. The other chief thrust towards a positive identity for the mentally ill is within the 'romantic tradition'. For example, R.D. Laing has proclaimed for 'the Schizophrenic as Saint', describing him as 'a Messiah bringing a message of truth for all of us'[54] Bateson views the psychotic experience as an opportunity for personal growth: 'a voyage of discovery.....(from) which he comes back with insights different from those inhabitants who never embarked on such a voyage'.[55] However, within

Western society sufferers of mental illness have proclaimed their creative uniqueness in works of art and literature which, as fields of individual endeavour, do not offer many opportunities for the promotion of solidarity.[56]

Summary

It has been a difficult task unravelling the major strategies used by patients to explain their hospitalisation in terms acceptable to themselves. One of the abiding features has been an acceptance of the benefits of the sick role as long as the self can be protected. It has been seen that there is a tension between the temporary gains of relief from responsibilities and the strains of filling the psychiatric patient role with its negative status and attendant stigma. The strategies which patients adopt to resolve this dilemma have an important feedback effect in facilitating or obstructing the return of the individual to the outside world.

Notes

1. Scheff, T. (1966) *Being Mentally Ill*, London.
2. Nunnally, J. (1961) *Public Conceptions of Mental Health*, New York. Nunnally found that the public depicted mentally ill patients as 'worthless', dirty, dangerous, cold, unpredictable and insincere' and he described them as wearing a 'negative halo'.
   Olmsted, D. and Durham, K. (1976) 'Stability of Mental Health Attitudes: A Semantic Differential Study', *Journal of Health and Social Behaviour*, 17, pp. 35-44. The authors found that the public viewed patients as unpredictable and dangerous.
3. O'Mahoney, P. (1981) *Public, Professional and Patient Perceptions of the Mentally Ill*', (unpublished Doctoral Thesis, Trinity College, Dublin). O'Mahoney found some evidence of familiarity and understanding of the mentally ill amongst the Irish.
4. Downey, K. (1967) 'Public Images of Mental Illness', *Social Science and Medicine* 1, pp. 45-65. The author reported that people used a Freudian explanation of mental illness but portrayed mental illness in terms of moral symptoms. He suggested 'that the trend from older folk beliefs to modern scientific explanations is only partial'.
5. Nunnally, J. (1961) op. cit.
6. Berger, P. (1977) Towards a Sociological Understanding of Psychoanalysis' in *Facing up to Modernity*, London. Berger uses the term 'psychologism' to describe the invasion of everyday life by the terminology and interpretative schemes of psychoanalysis, particularly in the areas of sexuality, marriage and child-rearing.
7. Jones, L. and Cochrane, R. (1981) 'Stereotypes of Mental Illness: A test of Labelling Hypothesis', *International Journal of Social Psychiatry*, 27, pp. 99-107. The authors found the stereotype of the mentally ill that existed in Britain conformed to the category of schizophrenia.
8. Scheff, T. (1966), op. cit. p. 1. The author describes his purpose as 'to formulate a sociological theory relevant to the understanding of the condition of chronic mental disease'.
   Scheff, T. (1975) 'Schizophrenia as Ideology' in *Labelling Madness*, New Jersey.
9. O'Mahoney, P. (1981) op. cit.

10. Cumming, E. and Cumming, J. (1957) *Closed Ranks: An Experiment in Mental Health Education*, Massachusetts.
11. Star, S. (1955) 'The Public's Ideas about Mental Illness'. Paper to the Annual Meeting of the National Association of Mental Health; Indianapolis. This classic study found 'that only the most extremely disturbed behaviour was recognised as such, by the majority of respodnents, who tended to resist calling anybody mentally ill, and they did so only as a last resort'.
12. Lemert, E. (1981) 'Issues in the Study of Deviance'. *The Sociological Quarterly*, 22, pp. 285-305.
13. Parsons, T. (1952) *The Social System*, Chapt. 10, London.
14. Scheff, T. (1975) op. cit. p. 7. Scheff makes a somewhat artificial distinction between physical and mental illness in terms of the former being 'culture free processes that are independent of the public order' unlike the symptoms of the latter which are 'offences against implicit understandings of particular cultures'. However studies of illness behaviour have also shown how the medicalisation of problems of bodily ill-health is also culturally influenced.
15. Rotenburg, M. (1974) 'Self-labelling: A Missing Link of the Societal Reaction Theory of Deviance', *Sociological Review*, 22, pp. 335-354.
16. Mead, G. (1964) *Selected Writings*, Indianapolis.
17. Rotenburg, M. (1974) op. cit.
18. Warren, C. (1974) 'The Use of Stigmatising Labels in Conventionalising Deviant Behaviour', *Sociology and Social Research*, 58, pp. 303-11.
19. Innes, G. and Sharp, G. (1962) ' A Study of Psychiatric Patients in North-East Scotland', *Journal of Medical Science*, 108, pp. 447-56.
20. Mezey, A. and Evans, E. (1971) 'Psychiatric In-Patient and Out-Patients in a London Borough', *British Journal of Psychiatry*, 118, pp. 609-16.
21. Linn, E. (1961) 'Agents, Timing and Events Leading to Hospitalisation', *Human Organisation*, 20, pp. 92-8.
22. Rose, S. and Hawkins, J. (1977) 'Decision to Admit: Criteria for Admission and Readmission to a V.A. 'Hospital', *Archives General Psychiatry*, 34, pp. 418-21.
23. Parsons, T. and Fox, R. (1953) 'Illness, Therapy and the Modern American Family', *Journal of Social Issues*, 8, pp. 31-44.
24. Illich, I. (1976) *Limits to Medicine*, London. The author has written extensively about 'medical imperialism'.
25. Rosenburg, G. and Attison, L. (1977) 'Attitudes towards Mental Illness in the Working Class'. *Social Work in Health Care*, 3, pp. 77-87. The authors found that working class people are less amenable to 'psychotherapeutic intervention' than their more affluent counterparts.
26. Raphael, E. (1964) 'Community Structure and Acceptance of Psychiatric Aid', *American Journal of Sociology*, 69, pp. 340-50. The authors assert that greater use is made of psychiatric facilities in areas of loose structure which are permeable to innovation.
27. These examples are drawn from the study sample and include both relevant parts of the interview and case summaries.

28. Rosenblatt, A. and Mayer, (1974) J. 'The Recidivism of Mental Patients: A Review of Past Studies' *American Journal of Orthopsychiatry*', 44, pp. 697-706.
29. Raphael, E. et al. (1966) 'Social Processes and Readmission', *Social Problems*, 13.
30. Hammer, M. (1963) 'Influence of Small Social Networks as Factors in Mental Hospitalisation', *Human Organisation*, 22, pp. 243-51.
31. Such thinking is reflected in the 1986 Mental Health Order which specifically excludes the diagnostic categories of alcohol abuse and personality disorder from compulsory admission to mental hospital.
32. Robinson, K. and Savage, M. (1985) 'Some Characteristics of Attempted Suicide Admitted to a District General Hospital', D.H.S.S. *Occasional Papers*, Belfast.
33. Kessel, N. and Lee, E. (1962) *'Attempted Suicide in Edinburgh, Scotland, Scottish Medical Journal*, 7, pp. 130-4. The authors describe a picture of 'preponderantly married women whose marital conflict is the chief aetiological factor...rather than social isolation as found by Sainsbury for suidice, it was not the lack but the explosiveness of personal relationships that is the significant factor'.
34. Furness, J., Khan, M. and Pickens, P. (1985) 'Unemployment and Parasuicide in Hartlepool 1974-1983', *Health Trends*, 17, pp. 21-24.
35. Giovanni, J. and Ullman, L. (1963) 'Conceptions of Mental Health by Psychiatric Patients, *Journal of Clinical Psychology*, 19, pp. 398-400.
36. Manis, M., Houts, P. and Blake, J. (1963) 'Beliefs about Mental Illness as a Function of Psychiatric Status and Psychiatric Hospitalisation', *Journal of Abnormal and Social Psychology*, 67, pp. 226-33.
37. Ibid.
38. Brady, J., Zeller, W. and Renzikoff, M. (1959) 'Attitudinal Factors influencing Outcome of Treatment of Hospitalised Patients'. *Journal of Clinical and Experimental Psychopathology*, 20, pp. 326-33.
39. Jones, N. and Khan, M. (1964) 'Patient Attitude as related to Social Class and other Variables concerned with hospitalistion', *Journal of Consulting Psychology*, 28, pp. 403-8.
40. O'Mahoney, P. (1981) op. cit.
41. Goffman, E. (1961) *Asylums: Essays on the Social Situation of Mental Patients and Other Inmates*, New York.
42. Ibid.
43. Cohen, S. and Taylor, L. (1972). *Psychological Survival*, London.
44. Quadagno, J. and Antonio, R. (1975) 'Labelling Theory as an Oversocialised Conception of Man; the Case of Mental Illness', *Sociology and Social Research*, 60, pp. 33-45.
45. Ibid, p. 43.
46. Goffman, E. (1961) op. cit.
47. Bateson, G. (1972) 'The Cybernetics of Self: A theory of Alcoholism', in *Steps to an Ecology of Mind*, London.
48. Bean, P. (1980) *Compulsory Admissions to Mental Hospitals*, p. 119, London.
49. Kennard, D. and Clemny, R. (1976) 'Psychiatric Patients as seen by Self and Others: an Explanation of Change in a Therapeutic Setting', *British Journal of Medical Psychology*, 49, pp. 35-53.

50. Goffman, E. (1961) op. cit.
51. Parsons, T. and Fox, R. (1953) op. cit.
52. Ibid.
53. Ellis, A. (1961) *The Rack*, Harmondsworth. This is a compelling account of the social life and growth of solidarity in a Swiss T.B. Sanatorium.
54. Laing, R. (1972) *The Politics of Experience*, London.
55. Bateson, G. (1974) *Perceval's Narrative: a Patient's Account of his Psychosis*, 1830-32, New York.
    Barnes, M. and Berke, J. (1971) *Mary Barnes: Two Accounts of a Journey through Madness*, London. This is an account of a psychotic experience by a patient and her psychiatrist from an existential standpoint.
56. There are plenty of examples of such individuals: for example, Dostoyevsky, Van Gogh and Graham Greene.

5 The family

In the previous theoretical discussion, the limits of a positive sociological approach have been outlined and the present research has come down in favour of a more ethnomethodological and interpretative approach. In the following discussion of the role of the family in the process of psychiatric hospitalisation, it is therefore the latter approach that is predominatly used.

In what follows there will be first an examination of the importance of the family in the referral process and the particular roles that the family fills in this respect. I then intend to examine the effects of family structural characteristics such as network, class and attitude on the labelling of mental illness, and compare my results with previous research. The second part of this chapter will be devoted to illustrating the activities of families as definers and labellers in order to highlight the dynamics of the process of psychiatric hospitalisation, and the strategies which families use in their efforts to come to terms with the behaviour confronting them.

The family setting is crucial and the activities of relatives are critical in the social process of interpretation and re-interpretation of disruptive behaviour as evidence of mental illness. Nearly one in three of the present sample were referred by relatives who were the first person to take effective action. This proportion is similar to the pattern found in other studies.[1]

The role of family members is essentially threefold. In the first place, interactionally, they experience, at first hand, all the major disruptions and also the small signs and acts that indicate that a person is not behaving according to prevailing norms. The consequences of unexpected and disturbing behaviour are a disruption of normal, everyday family routines such as eating, sleeping, home management and school and work attendance.[2]

If we are to examine the way in which social processes within the family culminate in hospital admission, we must look at the way in which mental symptoms disrupt social relations, the accommodations that are made towards them, and the strategies that are adopted by families in their efforts to cope with their consequences. Goffman has eloquently described the organisational havoc caused by episodes of manic behaviour,[3] and Lemert suggests that such speeded up, group-disruptive behaviour is potentially more likely to lead to hospitalisation than the seclusive behaviour of the schizophrenic.[4] Goffman quite rightly criticises sociologists for ignoring the consequences of disturbed behaviour when they have treated mental illness purely as a labelling process.[5]

The vulnerability of the nuclear family to disruption from illness behaviour has been emphasised by Parsons. He describes the sick role as a semi-legitimate means of withdrawal into a state of inactivity and dependance which requires care outside the family because of both the family's lack of resources and in order to minimise the risk of contaminating the 'motivational balance'.[6]

The second role of the family is as judge, to decide if changes in behaviour are unacceptable. Relatives will engage in a process of interpretation and re-interpretation of behaviour and use a variety of strategies in their attempts to deal with such behaviour. Research has shown that the imposition of the label of mental illness occurs only as a last resort when all other coping strategies have failed.[7] The stage at which this happens is not just governed by the recognition of the symptoms of mental illness by the family, but is also determined by the fact that the family is no longer able to cope, or is no longer prepared to tolerate the behaviour in question.[8]

Two research approaches have been adopted in analysing this process of decision making and re-interpretation. The first concentrates on the final act, the 'last straw' which makes the family petition for hospital admission.[9] The second is a more continuous approach that views the composition of the total picture of behaviour in terms of the 'accumulation of many inexplicable actions and statements'.[10] It is in this activity that the family act as arbiters and definers of what constitutes mental illness in the community. People arrive in hospital on the basis of these lay definitions of their behaviour. Families make ascriptions on the basis of 'untechnical', commonsense competence and the professional uses his technical competence to ratify these ascriptions.[11]

The third function of family members is to initiate action on the basis of their assessment and seek outside help. This is not straightforward; Clausen and Yarrow found that 'discontinuities and blocks to effective action were the rule rather than the exception...(and) many efforts to find a solution only led to 'dead-ends'.[12]

Enlisting outside professional help has been portrayed by Goffman as the betrayal of confidences and dishonouring of family allegiances.[13] Goffman described this process as the weaving of a 'collusive net' by which the definition of the situation is secretly managed by the colluders (relatives and doctors) against the 'excolluded' (the patient). Whilst the patient is made aware of the fact that his relatives are talking to hospital staff about him, he is unable to control what is being said, to what use such information is put, or how it is interpreted.

Structural Family Variables

Thomas Scheff emphasises the crucial importance of the availability of alternative forms of deviance and non-deviance in determining whether a person is labelled as mentally ill.[14] The availability of such alternatives is influenced by the structural characteristics of the family. These include the significance of the individual family network and the influence of social class on family attitudes. Both these factors help to determine the visibility of the offending behaviour. The tolerated parameters of 'mentally ill' behaviour within families are not fixed or stable but vary according to such structural characteristics.

A good deal of recent research has been geared to the development of the concept of social network to measure the availability of social, material and emotional support to the individual.[15] Attempts have been made to quantify particular characteristics of social networks in terms of their interconectedness or density. However, such research makes the rather simplistic assumption that human contact automatically means social support and that the closer the contact, the greater the support gained.[16] This ignores the potential for stress in close social contacts.[17]

The type of social network influences the availability of knowledge about mental illness and the methods of seeking professional help. It has been suggested that close kinship networks inhibit access to such information and services which results in delayed treatment.[18] The significance or importance of the person in the family has been cited as an important factor. However, it is unclear whether filling such roles as family breadwinner or primary-carer lead to delay in seeking help because of their importance, or speed up referral because of the increased visibility of the individual when performing these roles.[19]

Visibility is a crucial factor which has been linked to class membership mediated through attitudes. Myers and Roberts argue that within lower socio-economic families there is less inclination to view disturbed behaviour as mentally ill and consequently a delay in seeking treatment.[20] Other research emphasises the importance of social class in terms of the number of roles filled by the individual and suggests that individuals from higher socio-economic groups fill more roles so that changes in behaviour are more visible and require a more immediate response.[21] One of the chief difficulties with such research is that it requires some measure of duration of symptoms. In this study evidence is provided by retrospective accounts, but the identification of critical incidents is inevitably somewhat subjective.

Withdrawal is an important strategy adopted by individuals and families in their attempts to deal with changes in behaviour. It has been found that three-quarters of families with a schizophrenic relative experienced social withdrawal by that relative.[22] Families themselves will use secrecy, concealment and withdrawal in their attempts to cope.[23] The quality of family relationships has also been investigated as a determining factor although, as with all this research, there is a fundamental problem in identifying the independent variable.[24] As was detailed in an American study of depressed women,[25] deterioration in marital relationships may well be caused by the change in behaviour resulting from depression. But there is of course, a strong body of research which views family relationships as a pathogenic factor in mental illness.[26]

Research into structural family variables has also investigated the effect of such factors in influencing and predicting successful reintegration into family and community life.[27] In the present study, such structural factors as social class and significance in family networks are examined in order to assess their influence on hospital admission.

The literature on social class suggests that lower socio-economic groups delay seeking psychiatric help because they fear, are ignorant of, and deny mental illness. When hospitalisation occurs lower class patients are likely to display more aggressive and disturbed behaviour which is, in turn, likely to require compulsory admission to hospital.[28] This is not the case with my sample (see Appendix Three). A social class breakdown of formal admissions shows a distribution that compares with the social class breakdown of the sample as a whole. This finding conforms with a Chinese study which also reported no direct connection between threatening and aggressive behaviour and compulsory admission.[29]

Measurement of the significance of family role is difficult and analysis of the family processes involved may well be speculative. An indication of such factors is provided by a breakdown of the patient group referred by family, according to relative crucially involved (N = 53). (see Appendix Four). Spouses represent the largest single group of referrers amongst relatives as a whole. In the interpretation of these figures, living arrangement must also be considered. A quarter of those referred by relatives were involved with a partner in caring for children. This fact, together with the finding that spouses are the biggest referral group, would indicate, as expected, that child-care responsibilities are a crucial factor in the decision-making about hospitalisation. However, whether such child-care responsibilities hasten or delay admission cannot be conclusively established.

This has been a rather cursory interpretation of two family structural factors in a positive sociological mould. Whilst some researchers would argue that statistical analysis could untangle the relative significance of differing factors, my own research interest is with a move back into the actual content of family activity to highlight the behaviours involved and the strategies adopted by families in their attempts to cope.

An Ethnomethodological Approach

My approach towards mental illness and the family is concerned with the description of the minutiae of events occurring within the family and not the identification and isolation of particular variables. Such data-collection is inevitably retrospective as, it is obviously impossible to identify in advance those families who will utilise the mental illness label to deal with the behaviour they are experiencing, or to observe the build up of changes in actions and statements as they take place. Relatives, like everbody, need to make sense of their experiences and a process of 'backward reasoning' occurs in which particular past events are emphasised and reconstructed. This enables families to explain present labelling as the culmination of a chronological sequence of past behaviours and its logical outcome.[30]

Retrospective accounting by relatives has been used in previous studies of family processes and mental illness labelling. Such studies are, however, few and far between and the most important work remains that completed in the mid-fifties at the National Institute of Mental Health, Washington. This pioneering work was published in a series of articles which will be drawn upon in the following discussion of family coping strategies.[31] More recent work in this field has been completed under the auspices of the National Schizophrenic Fellowship, and is concerned with the strains of living with a schizophrenic relative.[32] Family effort to deal with identified behaviour is a dynamic process in which each effort to cope can be conceptualised as a process of adaptation. Each coping strategy is likely to influence the problem behaviour, either by successful adaptation in reducing it to acceptable norms, or by maladaptation when the problem behaviour is exaggerated or transformed into a further piece of problem behaviour. We have already seen in the previous chapter how this process takes place within the individual by self-interaction. We will now turn to the strategies adopted within families.

Family life, like other areas of social activity, is governed by a system of social rules and obligations. Infractions of such rules are challenged in an effort to modify rule-breaking behaviour and to influence the rule-breaker to return to behaving acceptably. If such efforts to modify behaviour are ineffective, the accommodation to the changed behaviour is likely to be the smallest necessary.[33] The family will constantly interpret and re-interpret behaviour as varying definitions are made and different coping strategies mobilised. As the level of problem behaviour varies so will the interpretations and strategies. A gradual movement towards a mental illness label may well take place but the label is only likely to be used as a last resort. Quiet periods will encourage momentary acceptance, normalisation and denial of previously unexplained and disruptive behaviour.

Charlotte Schwartz suggests that the process of defining of deviant behaviour in the family has a natural history.[34] At first, problem behaviour is likely to be ignored or denied. At which point behaviour is defined as problematic is likely to be determined by situational factors such as the personalities of those involved, the family value system, and the social supports available. Early interpretations of behaviour seem to be organised around explanations such as physical illness and stressful factors. When no ready explanation is available, behaviour may be viewed as accidental. Alternatively, it may be rationalised such as 'he's been working too hard', - or normalised such as 'he's going through an adolescent phase'. Strategies that go with such explanations are likely to use common-sense reasoning drawn from everyday life. Another early explanation may be organised around 'character problems'. A moralistic approach is then adopted in which behaviour is considered bad, wrong or sinful and in-laws or upbringing blamed such as 'he was always spoilt'. Such reactions are likely to be belligerent, recriminating and even threatening.

The pattern of labelling is influenced by the level of emotional attachment between labelled and labelee. It is to be expected that between marital partners there are considerable feelings of affection and loyalty which have to be overcome as well as feelings of guilt before outside help is sought.

Strategies that may be adopted in such circumstances include 'forcing the fit' by ignoring those aspects of behaviour that do not fit the interpretation made; 'balancing ' acceptable behaviour with unacceptable; and 'redefining the norms' by asserting that 'everyone's crazy these days'. The extent to which relatives are required to make such reinterpretations is influenced by the degree to which acts of deviant behaviour are visible and directly experienced in the family.

Finally, some researchers have interpreted hospital admission as a result of unresolved conflict in the family. Lemert originally spoke of 'spurious deviation' to describe situations of intra or inter-group struggle.[35]

Hospitalisation may also be seen as a demand for a change in behaviour,[36] or may be used by the 'ex-colluded' to show his preparedness to change. The importance of the sick role in placing responsibility for behaviour outside the individual into an illness symptomatology, facilitates and enables the individual's return to his family.

Critical Incidents and Problem Behaviours

Any attempt to quantify the behaviour in question is a somewhat arbitrary and subjective process. Some researchers have emphasised the importance of a particular incident which is viewed as the 'last straw' for the family who are then unable or no longer prepared to tolerate the perpetrator.[37] However before this, there is usually a whole build-up of changes in behaviour which in themselves may be relatively insignificant but which together go towards the decision to label mental illness. Admission to psychiatric hospital often occurs as an emergency and the 'backward reasoning' undertaken by relatives involves a re-interpretation of behaviours and events going back months and even years. The reliability of relatives' accounts may be questioned but the purpose is not so much the pursuit of some absolute truth as a description of the strategies, reasoning and explanations that families use to justify their actions and decision-making. In the present research I have used the concept of critical incident to define and divide the problem behaviours experienced by families. The number of categories of behaviour used is clearly of importance; for example, Whitmer and Conover identifed thirteen categories of incidents precipitating hospitalisation,[38] although their largest category included 'physicians's advice' which in this study is dealt with separately in the following chapter. Previous research would suggest that some form of violent or fear-inspiring behaviour is an important precipitating factor in a significant number of admissions.[39] Previous research has also distinguished between violent and grossly bizarre behaviour and other forms of behaviour.[40] In the present study I have divided the sample into three broad categories of problem behaviours.

Table 5.1: Patient Sample according to Problem Behaviour for Others

Problem behaviour	No. of incidents	%	Total
i) Disruptive			
Social nuisance	12	7)	
Aggressive/Threatening	21	12)	22
Breaking codes/laws	6	3)	
ii) Loss of reality/ self neglect			
Strange, bizarre thoughts	15	8)	
Withdrawn	17	9)	29
Self neglect/at risk	22	12)	
iii) Self-destructive			
Self-destructive/ suicidal	33	18))	38
Heavy drinking	36	20)	
iv) Other behaviours			11

Eight problem behaviours can be grouped into three broad categories. 'Self-destructive' is the largest of these accounting for 38% of problem behaviours as compared with only 11% in the Whitmer/Conover study. In this category are included not only suicidal acts, which represent the traditional imagery of mental illness, but also self-destructive behaviour through alcohol addiction. The second group of behaviours - 'loss of reality' and 'self-neglect' - accounts for 29% of behaviours as compared with a figure of only 16% in the Whitmer/Conover study in Utah. However the Desroches Canadian study reported a figure of 27%, similar to that of this study. This group covers the traditional symptomatology of mental illness. Disruptive behaviour accounts for 22% of the sample which compared with a figure of 10% in the Whitmer/Conover study. It should be said that such comparisons should be cautiously interpreted as the number of categories of behaviour varies between studies. A final category of 'other behaviours' accounts for 11% of incidents and includes exaggeration of personality and hospital contingencies. For example, in one instance, the psychiatrist was going on holiday and a troublesome patient was admitted in case she should cause difficulties whilst the doctor was away.

Case examples will be provided from each category of problem behaviour to show the social process of definition and the coping strategies used by families. Attention has already been drawn to the fact that problem behaviours overlap so that within each category other behaviours may also be in evidence.

i) Disruptive Behaviour

The behaviour subsumed under the present heading ranges from shouting and actual physical violence, throwing a brick through a window, and holding up traffic in the street to less overtly aggressive disruptions such as not sleeping at night and disturbing others by playing the record player too loud. Here are two examples describing the organisational havoc created and the family response to it.

> 'A' is a family man, living on state benefit for a number of years. Out of the blue, he started a business and used all his savings. The business failed and he ended up fighting with a customer and hurt his own head. At home, he began acting oddly; talking of his father not being dead and hearing his voice. He wrote notes about the rest of the family but when his wife reasoned with him, he said he was 'testing them' and got angry. She sought to hide his strange behaviour from the children. 'A' went out a great deal, drank heavily, spending recklessly and sometimes even tore up his money. His wife tried to influence his behaviour by accompanying him on his outings. 'A' lost weight and could not sleep. His wife cooked special meals for him but one night he accused her of not telling him that his children were dead. He threw his dinner across the room and his wife escaped to a neighbour's house. His wife rang for a doctor and a formal admission was arranged.

This case example can be analysed on a number of levels. In the first place, 'A''s changed behavour may be seen as a demand for a change in a marital relationship in which he was dependent and protected by his wife who was the main bread-winner. The nature of 'mentally ill' behaviour is clearly influenced by the nature of the marital relationship.[41] Mrs 'A' tolerated such changes at first but then sought to conceal them from the rest of the family and community. When 'A' made his behaviour more visible in the community, his wife sought to deny and normalise it. She resorted to explanations of physical illness (head injury) and overwork, when such behaviour could no longer be denied. She colluded with her neighbours in their social disapproval until the situation at home became intolerable. The 'last straw' was an act of unpredictable physical violence which resulted in compulsory hospitalisation. Whilst 'A' had been creating a significant amount of organisational havoc, it was not until he was openly violent that the 'mental illness' label was resorted to.

There are similiar characteristics in this second example.

> 'B' is an unemployed young man who lived with his parents. He has already been a patient at the Day Hospital, after becoming very timid and accompanying his mother everywhere. Back home, he has reverted to his outgoing self, only more so. 'B' stayed out

all night, but refused to tell his parents his whereabouts, and there were major family arguments. 'B' swore loudly at his parents in the middle of the street. They backed up their remonstrances by threatening him with the police who they called to 'have a talk with him'. These efforts were to no avail and his father wanted to throw him out of the home but his mother insisted he be allowed to stay. She argued that his behaviour was only 'a phase'. 'B' continued to disrupt family routines, playing loud music, watching T.V. as he wanted, and ordering the rest of the family to do as he said. His father was no longer prepared to tolerate him and there was a fight when 'B' hit his father. A doctor was called and his parents emphasised other aspects of 'B's behaviour: his muttering to himself; his Paracetomal taking; his rocking and staring; and his walking up and down. However, because it was the week-end the duty doctor refused to act until the family doctor returned who subsequently arranged formal admission two days later.

Again in this case, there may well have been an attempt by the perpetrator to bring about a change in family relationships which was not accepted by the rest of the family. B's confronting of his parents can be seen as a demand to be treated as an adult which was rejected by them. At first, they interpreted his behaviour as an adolescent phase but as B attempted to dominate and exercise control, the situation became intolerable for his parents. They called in outside help, resorting first to the police and a definition of delinquency, then they petitioned for medical help and a mental illness definition. Aggression was only the culmination in a whole series of behaviours which had been tolerated, rationalised and explained away. As Yarrow et al suggests, the family can be seen to posssss 'a monumental capacity to overlook, minimise and explain away evidence of profound disturbance in an intimate'.[42]

Location of behaviour is a crucial factor which has been conceptualised by Goffman in the phrase 'insanity of place'.[43] In these case examples, behaviour occurs in a family setting and relatives are involved in defining activities. However, when the perpetrator lives alone, changed behaviour is likely to come to attention as a social emergency involving social agencies as labellers.[44]

ii) Loss of Reality /Self Neglect Behaviours

Within this category is included the classic symptomatology of mental illness: hearing voices, experiencing delusions, confusion and withdrawal. What is crucial is how these behaviours impinge on and restrict the individual from fulfilling his normal role responsibilities.

'C' is the mother of young children, recently out of work and has become more and more concerned about paying the mortgage. She was not sleeping, unable to concentrate on the T.V. and worried about everybody's problems. Her husband worked long hours and

> enlisted the help of his mother in looking after 'C', and the children. 'C' dwelt in the past and talked of her childhood. She did not celebrate her wedding anniversary and became completely obsessed by the television news. She talked incessantly of the film 'The Exorcist' and reported a religious conversion; 'that the Devil has left me and God has entered my heart'. At the same time, she refused to leave the house and spent all her time looking out of the window. Her husband couldn't leave her and contacted his doctor for help, who arranged admission.

The relationship in this case is somewhat similar to that described by Sampson et al as the 'uninvolved husband and separate worlds'.[45] Husband's response initally was to involve his mother and, thereby, in some sense, increasing C's sense of isolation; she responded by not celebrating her wedding anniversary. Environmental factors were emphasised (financial pressure) as conventional explanations for her odd behaviour and her mother was brought in to help out 'C' who is' off form'. 'C' was searching for her own explanations and concentrated on her own childhood experiences as a cause for the way she felt. Her husband supported her in this explanation.[46] 'C' then looked for explanations outside herself and experienced a religious conversion which may be viewed as her own attempt at a coping strategy. Increasingly, relatives couldn't contain the situation demanding the full-time involvement of 'C's husband until the point was reached when she was clearly no longer able to care for the children and her social support network felt 'something must be done'.

In the present study, social withdrawal was a significant form of problem behaviour, a finding reported in other studies.[47] Social withdrawal may have the important function of concealing other changes in behaviour, not simply for the perpetrator but also for his family. But the isolated individual and family are left with less support to draw upon in times of crisis.[48] This lack of support may restrict access to alternative interpretations of behaviour and leave the family with only the mental illness label.

> 'D' is a middle-aged woman who lives with her mother. For many years she believed that she had a special relationship with God who controlled all her actions and decisions. She referred all matters to him and visited church frequently, believing that He spoke to her through the holy pictures in her house. However, there were times that she doubted her belief and believed that she was being taken over by the Devil. Her doubts were reinforced by her mother who sought to reason her out of her religious preoccupations. There were frequent arguments between them when her mother became angry with her. 'D' responded by retreating to her room for days at a time where she could be heard talking to herself. She returned to hospital, after coming to the Out-Patient Clinic to request alternative accommodation.

This example demonstrates how the relative's attempts at reasoning may exacerbate the situation. D's mother was elderly and had few social supports to draw upon. Hospitalisation offered an alternative during which relationships could be repaired and tolerance rebuilt. Admission may be viewed as a demand for removal from the deadlock that existed in family relationships. Willingness to enter hospital may demonstrate to one's family a recognition of their demands to change behaviour and a readiness to do so.

iii) Self Destructive Behaviour

Within this category are subsumed real suicidal threats, para-suicidal gestures, alcohol abuse and drug abuse. Whilst suicidal activity is seen as part of traditional mentally ill behaviour, the phenomenon of para-suicide (also known as 'non-deliberate self-harm or self-poisoning') is of more recent origin.[49] A recent study has associated such behaviour with married women aged under 25, with relationship problems. Such individuals often have no one with whom to confide and have been drinking before harming themselves impulsively.[50] In contrast, completed suicide is commoner among men than women, the elderly rather than the young, and amongst the single and unemployed. An example of each type of activity is presented.

> 'E' had not been sleeping well which had affected his performance at work. He attended his G.P. who treated him for tension and anxiety and environmental causes were emphasised. He began attending church regularly and became increasingly preoccupied with religious issues, believing that he had sinned. He did not find spiritual reassurance and his fears developed further and he feared he might be crucified. Believing that crowds of people were coming for him in the middle of the night, he ran out of the house, not returning till morning. His wife followed him but concealed his behaviour as she was afraid to tell anyone. One of 'E's earlier coping strategies had been heavy drinking which had created strains. Finally, one night 'E' called on his minister to speak to him but he was not at home. He became so desperate that he harmed himself and was treated at casualty. The next morning his wife rang their minister who confirmed the need for medical help and the G.P. was contacted who arranged admission.

There are a number of themes in this case. In the first place, E's attempts to cope became part of the problem. His drinking became alcohol abuse and his religious observance became religious delusion. This is a dynamic process involving feedback between problem behaviour and coping strategy when such strategies themselves are incorporated into problem behaviours. The second theme is the way in which his family tolerated a high degree of disturbance for fear of reprisals from 'E'. Only when physical self-harm could not be ignored was outside help enlisted by relatives. It can be seen that, as with other cases, the nature of family relationships was crucial in determining the pattern of events.

The second example is concerned with alcohol abuse and attempted suicide.

> 'F' is a mother addicted to alcohol over a number of years. Her husband took over the management of the home not allowing 'F' any money. In order to buy alcohol, she forged cheques, sold things from the home and drank perfume and meths. Previously, her husband regarded her as responsible for this behaviour which he saw as wilful and reacted to with violence. However, his actions did not modify her behaviour. Her husband redefined 'F's behaviour as illness when she returned home bruised and sick after a drinking binge. He persuaded her to see a doctor but neither 'F' nor the G.P. were anxious to medicalise her behaviour. The husband himself then recounted to the G.P. her past behaviour emphasising how she had attempted suicide. The doctor was persuaded to arrange admission to which 'F' was forced to agree as a condition for later returning home.

Although 'F' was no longer needed to care for the children, her drunken presence in the home created problems. It was the consequences of her disruptive behaviour and the need to ensure the survival of the family that demanded action. In this case, it can be seen how a relative may take a leading role in re-interpreting behaviour and defining it as 'mentally ill'. Pressures from relatives may well be the most significant factor in determining G.P. referral. The advantages of the illness definition in facilitating 'F's return to the family and enabling relationships to be repaired are clear-cut.

Summary

In the present chapter, attention has been concentrated on the strategies adopted within families, each of which has a label of deviance or non-deviance attached. The nature of such labels will be influenced by the cultural context and some of those which may be found in an Irish context are now suggested. Families may accept the care of a mentally ill relative and describe him as a 'a cross to bear'. This description indicates the spiritual support for long term suffering. Judgement of behaviour seems to take place along a continuum. Extreme behaviour is known as 'being as mad as a March hare'. Falling short of such labelling , points along the continuum are suggested by a whole variety of descriptions which carry a somewhat less attendant stigma. Some of these are :'not the full shilling'; 'a few bricks short of a load'; 'four sheets to the wind'. The family may conceal the problem which may be referred to as 'the skeleton in the cupboard'. 'The black sheep of the family' describes a convenient form of scapegoating in which the responsibility for all the family trouble is blamed on one person. Explanations of odd behaviour in terms of physical health use such phrases as 'a bit delicate' and 'bad with the nerves'.

The possibility or availability of alternative forms of deviance and non-deviance has been associated with some structural variables such as social class attitudes, social support networks and level of significance in families. Studies of illness behaviour have predictably emphasised tolerance or 'threshhold for seeking help' as a critical factor.[51] The level of tolerance is set by ideological factors such as attitude to health, and situational factors such as knowledge and access to medical services. What Goffman calls 'career contingencies' include proximity to mental hospital and availability of beds as well as socio-economic status and visibility of offence. Any suggested model of mental illness behaviour must take into account such contingencies.

Studies of patients with physical complaints have described four stages in illness recognition. These are: experience of pain or discomfort which may be emotionally disturbing; 'provisional validation' by describing to significant others and receiving agreement to suspend the sick person's normal obligations; professional legitimation of the sick role by consulting a doctor; and the doctor's response - his assumption of some internal disagreement and his prescription.[53] However, it is clear that the recognition of mental illness behaviour is not nearly so straightforward because it is often the case that the pre-patient does not recognise that anything is wrong. Even if he does, he may well see his problems in terms that are far removed from illness. The importance of the concept of 'insight' in accepting the mental illness label has been dwelt upon in the previous chapter.

In this respect, significant others, primarily the pre-patient's family, are of crucial importance. However, the role of the family extends beyond a sense of responsibility, which was one of the roles identified in the study of the management of illness in children.[54] Goffman has identified two distinct stages in the pre-patient phase: firstly, some offence against an arrangement of face to face living; and secondly, the effective move of recording some complaint which marks the social beginning of the patient's career (regardless of where one might locate the psychological begininning of his mental illness).[55] The moral career of the patient is then characterised by successive stages during which the individual's status is reduced and, by a psychiatric work-up of his past, his behaviour is reinterpreted in the light of his present status as psychiatric patient.

The betrayal aspects of this process have been emphasised and a model of exclusion is suggested. The interpretation and reinterpretation of behaviour within the family, with successive forms of deviance being identified until the label of mental illness is resorted to, may be seen as a downward spiral with the identified individual at the centre. Items of behaviour that his family find problematic may be coped with by strategies which bring about a further problematic response from the individual. Again, the family seeks to adapt and, by so doing, may cause an exaggeration of the problem behaviour or the addition of further difficulties. As this process of maladaptation proceeds, outsiders may be called upon to bring new definitions which consider the wider social consequences of the behaviour in question. Problematic behaviour in the family may become social trouble and the downward spiral accelerates. With hospitalisation the downward spiral continues as the individual takes on the stigma of the psychiatric patient role.

Notes

1. Lynne, E. (1961) 'Timing and Events leading to Mental Hospitalisation'. *Human Organisation*, pp. 92-8.
   Horowitz, A. (1978) 'Family Kin and Friend Networks in Pyschiatric Help-Seeking', *Social Science and Medicine*, 12, pp. 297-304.
   Rose, S. and Hawkins, J. (1977) 'Decision to Admit', *Archives General Psychiatry*, pp. 418-21.
2. Trudley, M. (1946) 'Mental Illness and Family Routines', *Mental Hygiene*, 30, pp. 235-40. The author describes the disruption of family routines from case records of hospital admissions.
3. Goffman, E. (1971) *Relations in Public, 'Insanity of Place*, London. The appendix contains an illuminating discourse on the repercussions of 'manic' behaviour.
4. Lemert, E. (1946) 'Legal Commitment and Social Control' in *Sociology and Social Research.*
5. Goffman, E. (1971) op. cit. p. 413.
6. Parsons, T. and Fox, R. (1953) 'Illness, Therapy and the Modern American Family', *Journal of Social Issues*, 8, pp. 31-44.
7. Clausen, J. and Yarrow, M. (1955) 'Paths to the Mental Hospital', *Journal of Social Issues*, 11, pp. 25-32.
8. Meyers, J. and Roberts, B. (1959) *Family and Class Dynamics in Mental Illness*, New York.
   Whitmer, C. and Conover, C. (1959) 'A Study of the Critical Incidents in the hospitalisation of the mentally ill'. *Journal of the National Association of Social Work*, 4, pp. 89-94.
9. Ibid.
10. Clausen, J. and Yarrow, M. (1955) op. cit.
11. Bastide, R. (1972) *The Sociology of Mental Disorder*, London.
12. Clausen, J. and Yarrow, M. (1955) op. cit.
13. Goffman, E. (1961) op. cit. Goffman describes a 'betrayal funnel':- 'Each stage brings a decrease in free status, while each agent tries to maintain a fiction. This is done in a seducing way to maintain harmony and avoid the patient dealing with the raw emotion he wants to express'.
14. Scheff, T. (1966) *Being Mentally Ill*, London.
15. Gottlieb, B. (1983) *Social Networks and Social Supports*. New York.
16. See for instance the work of Henderson, S., British Journal of Psychiatry, (1977-80).

17. Brown, G., Birley, J. and Wing, J. (1972) 'Influence of Family Life on the Course of Schizophrenic Disorders', *British Journal of Psychiatry*, 121, pp. 241-58.
18. Horowitz, A. (1977) 'Social Networks and Psychiatric Treatment', *Social Forces*, 56, pp. 86-104.
Raphael, E. (1964) 'Community Structure and Acceptance of Psychiatric Aid', (1964) *American Journal of Sociology*, 69, pp. 340-50.
19. Hammer, M. (1963) 'Influence of Small Social Networks as Factors in Hospitalisation', *Human Organisation*, 22, pp. 243-51.
20. Myers, J. and Roberts, B. (1959), op. cit.
21. Hammer, M. (1963) op. cit.
22. Creer, C. and Wing J. (1974) *Schizophrenia at Home*, Surbiton.
23. Yarrow, M., Clausen, J. and Robbins, P. (1955) 'The Social Meaning of Mental Illness', *Journal of Social Issues*, 11, pp. 33-48. The authors found that a third of wives whose husbands had been hospitalised demonstrated a pattern of aggressive concealment.
24. Sampson, H., Messinger, S. and Towne, R. (1962) 'Family Processes and becoming a mental patient', *American Journal of Sociology*, pp. 88-96.
25. Weissman, M. and Paykel, E. (1974) *The Depressed Woman: a Study in Social Relationships*, Chicago.
26. Lidz, T. (1957) 'Marital Schism and Marital Skew', *American Journal of Psychiatry*, pp. 241-8.
Bateson, G., Jackson, D., Haley, J. and Weakland, J. (1956) 'Towards a Theory of Schizophrenia' *Behavioural Science*, 1, pp. 251-64.
27. Freeman, H. and Simmons, O. (1959) 'Familial Expectations and Post-Hospital Performance of Mental Patients', *Human Relations*, pp. 233-41.
Denitz, S., Lefton, M. and Angrist, S. (1961) 'Psychiatric and Social Attributes as Predictors of Case Outcome in Pyschiatric Hospitalisation', *Social Problems*, 8.
28. Haney, C. and Miller, K. (1970) 'Definitional Factors in Mental Incompetence', *Sociology and Social Research*, 54, pp. 520-32.
29. Hsu, F. (1939) 'Police Co-operation in Connection with Mental Cases in Peiping' in *Neuro-psychiatry in China* (1939) eds. Lyman, R., Maeker, V. and Liang, P. From a somewhat different data base, this Chinese study suggested that families are most frequently concerned with thought-disordered behaviour.
30. Smith, D. (1978) 'K is mentally ill: the Anatomy of a Factual Account', *Sociology*, 12, pp. 23-53. This is a good example of this process.
31. Clausen, J. and Yarrow, M. (1955) 'The Impact of Mental Illness on the Family', *Journal of Social Issues*, 11, pp. 3-67.
32. Creer, C. and Wing, J. (1974) op. cit.
33. Hammer, M. (1963) op. cit.
34. Yarrow, M., Schwartz, C., Murphy, H. and Deasy, L. (1955) 'The Psychological Meaning of Mental Illness in the Family', *Journal of Social Issues*, 11, pp. 12-24.
Schwartz, C. (1957) 'Perspectives of Deviance', *Psychiatry*, XX, pp. 275-91.
35. Lemert, E. (1946) op. cit.

36. Woods, E., Rakusin, J. and Morse, M. (1960) 'Interpersonal Aspects of Psychiatric Hospitalisation', *Archives of General Psychiatry*, 3, pp. 632-41.
Polak, P.R., (1967) 'The Crisis of Admission' *Social Psychiatry*, 2, pp. 150-7.
37. Whitmer, C. and Conover, G. (1959) 'A Study of Critical Incidents in the Hospitalisation of the Mentally Ill'. *Journal of the National Association of Social Work*, IV, pp. 89-94.
38. Ibid.
39. Lagos, J., Perlmutter, K. and Saxinger, M. (1977) 'Fear of the Mentally Ill: Empirical Support for the Common Man's Response', *American Journal of Psychiatry*, 134, pp. 1134-37. They quote a figure of 36% of admissions being preceded by some incident of aggressive or fear inspiring behaviour.
Haney, C, and Miller, K. (1970) op cit. The authors found that between 42-48% of cases involved violence or aggression.
40. Desroches, F. (1980) *Mental Illness in the Family - the Decision to Enter Hospital*, (unpublished Ph.D dissertation, University of Waterloo, Canada, 1980) In a classification of patients' deviant behaviour, 48% of incidents of hostility and 57% of actual or potentially harmful behaviour were reported.
41. Sampson, E. et al (1962) op. cit. The authors describe two martial patterns of accommodation: the uninvolved husband and separated worlds; and the overinvolved mother and the marital family triad.
42. Yarrow, M. et al (1955) op. cit.
43. Goffman, E. (1971) op. cit.
44. Bean, P. (1980) *Compulsory Admissions to Mental Hospital*, London. The author reports that when the miscreant lived alone, social emergencies occurred which involved agencies like the police and social services.
45. Sampson, H. et al. (1962) op. cit. p. 44.
46. Schwartz, C. (1957) op. cit. This fits into the characterological framework which the author described as where difficulties are perceived as being due to something defective in character or personality.
47. Creer, C. and Wing, J. (1974) op. cit. Three quarters of the families interviewed stated that the social withdrawal of the schizophrenic was the most frequenjtly experienced problem.
48. Taylor, R., Huxley, P. and Johnson, D. (1984) 'The Role of Social Networks in the Maintenance of Schizophrenic Patients', *British Journal of Social Work*, 14, pp. 129-140. The authors report that good social performance of the patient is associated with wider patterns of social interaction for his relatives.
49. Kreitman, N., Philip, A., Greer, S. and Bagley, C. (1969) 'Para-suidice' *British Journal of Psychiatry*, 115, pp. 746-7.
50. Robinson, K. and Savage, M. (1985) 'Some Characteristics of Attempted Suicide Admitted to a General Hospital'. D.H.S.S., *Occasional Paper*, Belfast.
51. Kessel, N. and Shepherd, M. (1965) 'The Health and Attitudes of People who Seldom Consult a Doctor', *Medical Care*, 3, pp. 6-10.
52. Goffman, E. (1961) op. cit.

53. Goldberg, D. and Huxley, P. (1980) Mental Illness in the Community. p. 47, London.
54. Strong, P. (1979) *The Ceremonial Order of the Clinic*, London.
55. Goffman, E. (1961) op. cit.

6 The religious perspective and the informal network

According to the Scheffian position, the extent of use of the mental illness label as a category for explaining residual deviance is determined by the availability of alternative labels of deviance and non-deviance.[1] In the following chapters the activities of the main labellers are examined in turn. Each group has the possibility of mobilising its own descriptions of the behaviour presented to it. For instance, the police may view behaviour as criminal, whilst the family see it as wilful, and the clergyman describes it as sinful.

Historically, the behaviour subsumed under the term 'mental illness' has been dealt with in religious terms as 'the cure of souls'. Anthropological study of 'primitive' societies has attested to their continued use of such a perspective. The Polar Eskimos for example, believe that disease results from the loss of the soul.[2] Christian beliefs are outlined in the story of the man who said 'My name is Legion: for we are many'.[3] This man is described as crying and living amongst the tombs as 'no man could bind him, neither could any man tame him', a description of what now may be called schizophrenia. Jesus cleansed the man who had an unclean spirit by sending the spirits into a herd of swine who ran over a cliff into the sea.

Behaviour now viewed as 'mental illness' was seen in the Bible as a spiritual matter.[4] The importance of these accounts for Christians is their demonstration of the supreme powers of God through the work of Jesus Christ, the rewards of which are only possible for those who have faith in Him. Christians believe that such spiritual gifts are given to some amongst them and these spiritual powers include the gift to distinguish between spirits and to interpret 'tongues'.[5] These are the Biblical justifications that ministers invoke when they involve themselves with 'mentally ill' behaviour.

Thomas Ssasz, whilst bemoaning the neutralising of moral dilemmas by psychiatry, elaborates on the persecution of elderly women by religious bodies such as the Inquisition.[6] It seems probable that most of the women condemned as witches would be now regarded as psychotic[7] but in the Middle Ages belief in evil spirits flourished and exorcism was the therapeutic technique of choice.[8] With the rise of rationalism and the methods of science came also the 'period of great confinement' in the seventeenth and eighteenth centuries.[9] Institutions increasingly came under medical supervision in the nineteenth century and by the end of the century the psychiatric approach emerged supreme.

To what extent is it possible for the psychiatric and religious perspectives to be reconciled? Klausner has usefully applied Parsons' pattern variables to the differing norms and expectations that define the respective roles of ministers and psychiatrists.[10] In the first place, psychiatrists emphasise training and competence and hence are achievement-orientated whilst ministers respond to a 'call'and their role is 'ascriptive'. Secondly, a psychiatrist is 'specific' in his relationship with his patient whilst a minister is 'diffuse' in that his relationship extends to many situations. Thirdly, a psychiatrist stays 'affectively neutral' but a minister should give unconditional love and is 'affective'. Finally, the psychiatrist aims for a role that is 'universalistically orientated' since all patients are treated as opportunities for treatment; on the other hand, a minister is 'particularistic' in that a single relationship takes precedence over general rules. Finally, both are seen as being 'collectively orientated'.

In America, there are instances where clergy and doctors work alongside each other in religio-psychiatric clinics which use a counselling approach to deal with emotional problems. Such practitioners describe a 'Christian Psychiatry that reaches down into the soul and treats the whole man - spirit , soul, and body'.[11] The main tenets are those of fundamentalist Christianity: that 'it is impossible for a man not to sin because he is born alienated from God'; that 'God is part of the whole counselling process in that he has outlined in the Bible a way for individuals to bring their needs to Him'; and that spiritual regeneration is necessary to 'enter into a personal relationship with God'.[12] Christianity is seen as a root solution that reaches all levels of man.

Whilst the findings of American research cannot be simply applied to Northern Ireland there are certain similarities in the clergyman's role in both countries. The particular exigencies of the local scene will be returned to in more detail after a general discussion. It has been found in America that people with emotional problems most frequently seek help from a clergyman.[13] He is the first person to be approached but his involvement is often brief and because he is approached so early in the search for help, he is frequently called upon to allocate clients to other agencies.[14] Ministers are dissatisfied with this role since, whilst they refer many cases, there is little recipricocity.[15] Other research has suggested that ministers are well suited to offer help as they are nearest to their clients in terms of social distance, involvement in the community and mutual understanding.[16] Whether a minister does make a referral to a psychiatrist is influenced by his own socio-economic and educational background. Higher status, higher education and large congregations are characteristics of those clergymen closer to the psychiatric norms[17]. This finding is of particular significance to the Northern Ireland situation.

Northern Ireland is a society divided along religious lines. The consequences of this for everyday interaction is to make religion something of a taboo subject. This has strengthened the position of psychiatry operating in a rather traditional religious society. Psychiatry has also been able to to hold itself aloof from religious intervention. For example, referrals are not usually made by psychiatrists to clergymen. This may be because psychiatrists need to show themselves neutral towards religious loyalties although it is not clear to what extent such referrals are made elsewhere such as England. Sometimes, psychiatrists criticise ministers' moralising about patients conduct, and do not make referrals to clergymen for this reason.

The ministers I interviewed acted as hospital chaplains. One clergyman expressed his resentment at the hegemony of doctors, the fact that ministers were not invited to attend ward rounds, and that people were more prepared to talk openly to a doctor than a minister. On the other hand, another 'mainline' Protestant clergyman expressed satisfaction with a subordinate role and saw his role as one of reassurance and encouraging patients to take medical advice. These ministers thought of healing as God's work; doctors were seen as the instruments of the Supreme Healer. In general, like their American counterparts[18] they accepted their role. One of their concerns was the protection of their own flock against the activities of proselytizers; all watched for such activity and if observed, medical staff were called upon to ask such preachers to be prevented from visiting the hospital. In this activity, both doctors and clergy were united. The activities of evangelical Protestants are of particular interest as they clearly saw themselves as involved with behaviour which might be otherwise categorised as 'mentally ill'. Whilst the rhetoric of the major denominations recognises the presence of the Devil, in practice the main churches are much less willing than the evangelicals to recognise demon possession.

The evangelical churches have a number of religious techniques which are regularly used to deal with 'mentally ill' behaviour. Some of those diagnosed mentally ill had been taken by relatives to have hands 'laid on'. Relatives seemed able to accommodate the apparently contradictory religious and illness perspectives. Other healing practices include 'witnessing', when a person recounts how his faith has made him well, and is exhorted to pray harder and atone for sins. When attempted in the hospital such practices led to the banning of the minister from the hospital as described in the following case example.

> 'A' lived with her boyfriend and her family, who belonged to an Evangelical Church, disapproved. However, after a family death, 'A' became very religious and believed she was committing a sin by cohabiting. She felt she had to choose between God and her boyfriend and left her boyfriend to go back to her family. She still believed that she had sinned and attempted suicide. In hospital she was visited by her minister who emphasised that she had done wrong. The Pastor was banned from visiting anybody in the hospital, and reprimanded by the psychiatrist.

The psychiatrist dominates the hospital setting; he is likely to hold to a conventional attitude which keeps 'religion for Sunday' and to discourage frequent Bible study (particularly of the Book of Revelations!). The case of 'A' also shows the heavy demands on the individual that may be made by religion, demands which may in extreme case precipitate hospitalisation. A disproportionate number of members of evangelical churches were admitted as patients during the research period. The Evangelical churches accout for only 3% of the District population but 13% of the hospital admission sample. The socio-economic background of evangelical ministers has been offered as an explanation for their disagreement with psychiatry and psychiatrists.[19] But their lack of access to medical professionals is offset by their solidarity with their working class congregations. Clergymen are important as social supports and referral agents.

> Mrs 'B' had exasperated her family by her demands for their involvement. They sought to place limits on their contact and only saw her at regular intervals which were prearranged. Her neighbours also stopped giving her support for the same reason. Her family refused to visit when she phoned and Mrs 'B' went to her clergyman's house to seek help. When there was a scene in the street after her family refused to be involved in hospitalisation, her clergyman then contacted the G.P. who arranged admission.

There were two other instances of people seeking minister's help but in both cases they did not succeed in making contact. In one, the minister had proved a great source of help over many years. This is the nature of most clergymen's activity; although they are not usually part of the decision to seek medical help, they are generally supportive at other times. The church is a primary source of social support and much of that personal support comes from the minister. Clergy represent part of the informal network of support which functions independently of formal networks. American research has shown that they are particularly called upon to help people in situations of marital and family difficulties, and, in their intervention in this area, they are less likely to make referrals to other agencies.[21]

In Northern Ireland, there may well be differences between churches in their pastoral activity. Catholic clergy administering to large and diffused congregations seem to be primarily involved with the religious duties of their church and its congregation. 'Main-line' Protestant clergy may also have large congregations which limit their degree of involvement on an individual basis. In contrast, the evangelical churches, with one or two exceptions, represent small and loyal communities of interest. The following example shows the degree of support given.

> 'C' is a member of an evangelical sect. She attended Bible study and Church services three evenings a week and a Youth Club two evenings. 'C' phoned her minister and his wife every day and sometimes at night. They visited her in her flat and she confided first to her minister, rather than her mother.

Such strongly supportive ties are very important to individuals and are highly valued. That this is an ideal of support which others may envy is demonstrated by an elderly lady who fabricated a story of daily visits from her minister and nightly suppers at his home, instead of the reality of loneliness, too many tablets and too much drink.

The fact that clergy are not involved in referrals to psychiatric hospital may also be explained by the universal availability of health care. The clergyman does not act as a gatekeeper; a person's hospital admission can be effectively negotiated by family, neighbours and friends in contact with medical personnel. In one case, although the minister was present during the pre-hospital crisis, it was the neighbour who contacted the doctor to arrange admission. A second explanation for ministers' lack of involvement in the referral process may lie in the characteristics of church and church membership. The mainline churches with a clergy favourably disposed to psychiatry have large congregations which prevent them from being intimately involved in the decision-making of individual parishioners. On the other hand, those small churches with strong links between clergyman and congregation hold to an evangelical ideology which is broadly antipathetic to psychiatry. Finally, clergy have no formal powers and the use of coercion is incompatible with their pastoral role. For all these reasons, clergymen are rarely used in getting a reluctant patient into hospital.

Friends and neighbours are principally involved in the process of hospitalisation of a group of patients who are subsequently diagnosed as suffering from personality disorders. Neighbours are also involved with isolated people whose behaviour has made them unable to look after themselves. In several cases, neighbours and friends were very effective complainants in situations where the individual had been refused admission. Research into the operation of informal networks suggests that individuals are more likely to seek help with emotional problems from friends, and with material problems from their families [22]. On the other hand, it has also been suggested that friends and neighbours, being less emotiomally committed, are more likely to resort to the definition of mental illness.[23]

> Mr 'C' lived alone after his relative went into hospital and did not look after himself, drinking heavily. 'C' wanted to be readmitted to hospital but his doctor refused to see him because of his drinking. When 'C' could not eat or sleep, his neighbour arranged a taxi to take him to hospital. Admission was refused and he returned to his neighbour who contacted a local doctor to insist on his being admitted. A few weeks later when he was discharged he resumed drinking and his neighbour again insisted on her own doctor coming out to get him back into hospital.

It seems unlikely that a clergyman would become involved in such a situation or demand resolution to the same extent. His social distance prevents such involvement or intimate acquaintance with the informal ways of achieving help. Nor is he required to tolerate the disturbances of such behaviour at first hand, which would also increase his motivation to achieve removal. The minister thus stands apart from the rest of the informal helping network, constrained both by a religious ideology and by social distance which gives rise to a distinct set of norms and expectations.

Religion as Symptom

There is a widely held belief that psychiatric patients are preoccupied by religion. This has been challenged by the work of Lowe and Braaten who found that patients seem to exhibit less religious participation than those in the community.[24] This result may be explained by the deadening and isolating effects of institutional life which saps individual interest and motivation. The researchers found some support for this interpretation in the evidence of newer patients being more ready to use religion in an instrumental way. Nevertheless, in the present study religious topics are a matter of frequent concern for some patients. For example, one patient reported seeing the Devil coming out of the light bulb; another feared that people were coming to crucify him; a third believed that all her actions were ordered by God. What is of interest is the way patients were prepared to go along with the reinterpretation of their religious preoccupations as symptoms of mental illness. There was evidence of psychiatrists not confronting such contradictions so that patients were able to compartmentalise their beliefs.

> 'D' is a young mother whose children were in the care of Social Services and had returned to live with her parents. She believed for some time that a neighbour had put her under the control of the Devil. 'D' attended a gospel hall regularly and stated that since she had been baptised with the Holy Spirit, the Devil did not know when she spoke to God because she used a different language entirely. She stated that her neighbours probably thought she was mad when she spoke 'in tongues' because to them it would sound like gibberish.

'D's religious behaviour which was seen as illness in hospital was encouraged as evidence of her salvation when she was in her evangelical church. It was only when her social worker visited and found her 'withdrawn', in poor health, and neglecting herself that admission was initiated.

The strains of accommodating a religious perspective with psychiatric patient status are particularly marked for a patient who is a minister or missionary. What seems to occur is a holding in abeyance of religious practice which may call into question the basis of belief. One pastor patient commented that he saw examples of devilry in other patients, which he termed extra-terrestial activity, but was aware of his status of patient and held back from ministering to such cases. There are clearly obvious strains in accommodating the two perspectives.

A similar situation arises for staff with evangelical beliefs. As occurred with one new doctor, those who openly proselytise are quickly admonished and moved on to less visible work. However, such activity may be carried on unknown to the psychiatrist and arrangements made with the patient to attend prayer meetings after discharge. Thirdly, staff may argue for their beliefs but justify medical intervention to treat thought disorder, agitation, anxiety and other symptoms which prevent the patient from concentrating on a spiritual solution. Medicine is thus seen as making the person amenable to spiritual guidance.

It has been suggested that denominational affiliation may also influence the nature of psychiatric disturbance. An analysis of psychotic symptoms according to church membership found that one half of Protestants had delusions with a religious content as compared to one quarter of Catholics.[25] McDonald and Luckett divided Protestants into 'non-mainline ' and 'mainline' and found that the former had a high proportion of depression and the latter were dominated by personality disorders.[26] They also found that Catholics were obsessional and hysterical. However, research in Northern Ireland has shown an excess of schizophrenia in the never married Catholics.[27] Catholics are also twice as likely to be hospitalised for alcoholicism.[28]

It can be seen that religious practices are filtered through cultural background to influence the nature of psychiatric symptoms. Attempts to explain such relationships are largely conjectural. For instance, the preponderance of Catholic schizophrenics has been explained in a West of Ireland context by the 'persecution by ridicule' common in Irish conversation,[29] the power of Irish mothers over their sons reflected in a peculiar demographic structure of late marriage with high rates of female emigration,[30] and by a sense of relative deprivation.[31]

Table 6.1: Religious Affiliation and Psychiatric Diagnosis.

Religion Diagnosis District.		Schizo.	Affect.	Pers Dis.	Sample
	%	%	%	%	%
Religion/					
Church of Ireland	20	25	40	36	23
Presbyterian	18	30	35	26	33
Non-Conformist	8	12	65	10	13
Catholic	30	12	30	15	9
Evangelical	18	25	33	14	3

The above table shows that schizophrenia accounts for a larger proportion of diagnoses for Catholics than other religious groups. One possible explanation for this may be a lower rate of utilisation of state services by other Catholic diagnostic groups, particularly those subsumed under the heading personality disorders. The present study also supports the idea that Protestants are more prone to depression, which may be explained by the Protestant emphasis on sin and guilt. Evangelical churches, in particular, have high expectations of their members and thus give more opportunities to fail and more possibilities of guilt.

What is of particular interest is the large number of people categorised as personality disorders from the main Protestant churches. Given the low rate of church attendance already reported for these groups, their church membership is clearly nominal. People in this group are not in a position to interpret their behaviour in a religious framework and may be more likely to resort to the residual category of mental illness. Their alienation may be more acutely felt in the religious society of Northern Ireland. A similiar finding was reported in a similarly religious society, an American Mid-Western state with a high proportion of patients with 'no religious preference'.[32] Such persons are not likely to have a clergyman available to call in times of need, and this is another reason why clergmen are of only marginal interest in this discussion of routes to hospital.

Summary

Clergymen stand on the edge of the process of psychiatric hospitalisation. Whilst there is some evidence that they may act independently to provide social support systems which shore up vulnerable individuals, once behaviour is characterised as psychiatric they assume a subordinate role. The only exceptions are evangelical activists who, because of their religious beliefs and their absence of socioeconomic solidarity with doctors, may be prepared to contest the medical perspective. However, any discovered attempts to infiltrate the hospital system are squashed. Patients are likely to hold evangelical activity in abeyance whilst in hospital.

The extent to which religious preoccupation is interpreted as illness symptoms is related to the patient's pre-illness level of religiosity, as well as the theological standpoint of those doing the assessment. In general terms, religious preoccupations are likely to be used as evidence of symptoms in hospital. This is illustrated in the rule of thumb of one psychiatrist who saw feelings of having sinned as a very positive indicator for E.C.T. for patients diagnosed as suffering from depression.

The acquiescence of the clergy to the ideological supremacy of the medical model is an indication of their uncertainty in a secular world. The battle between religion and medicine was effectively won one hundred years ago by medicine and doctors have been characterised as the 'new priests'. However, in the field of mental illness, the boundaries between the secular and the spiritual remain blurred in a way that does not happen in physical medicine. This is because psychiatry is involved in making judgements about conduct, beliefs and values, things that had been previously the preserve of the church. Ministers have accepted psychiatry's sole legitimacy within the hospital. However, we are unable to say how far ministers make such judgements outside hospital, although research indicates that their role is limited.

Notes

1. Scheff, T. (1966) *Being Mentally Ill*, London.
2. Beals, R. and Hoijer, H. (1965) *An Introduction to Anthropology*, p. 583, London.
3. St. Mark, Chapt. V., verses 1-16.
4. Matthew, Chapt. 17, verses 14-18: this passage describes an epileptic boy having a demon cast out. Mark, Chapt. V, verses 25-34 reports a woman being cured of a haemorrhage. John, Chapt. IX, verses 1-8 describes a man born blind, made to see (his blindness is explained by the disciples as due to he or his parents having sinned).
5. Corinthians I, Chapt. XII, verse 10.
6. Szasz, T. (1972) *The Myth of Mental Illness*, St. Albans.
7. Mora, G. (1975) 'Historical and Theoretical Trends in Psychiatry' in *Comprehensive Textbook of Psychiatry*, edited by Friedman et al, Vol 1, Baltimore.
8. Clausen, J. and Hufine, C. (1975) 'Socio-Cultural and Socio-Psychological Factors affecting Social Response to Mental Disorder', *Journal of Health & Social Behaviour*, 16, pp. 405-20.
9. Foucault, (1976) *Madness and Civilisation*, New York.
10. Klausner, S. 'Role and Adaptations of Pastors and Psychiatrists'.
11. Little, G. (1970) *The Christian and Emotional Problems*, Nebraska.
12. Cosgrave, M. and Mallory, J. (1977) *Mental Health: A Christian Approach*, Michigan.
13. Gurin, G., Veroff, J. and Field, S. (1960) *Americans View Their Mental Health*, New York. It was found from a nationwise sample that 42% of people with emotional problems first saw a clergyman.
14. Cummings, E. and Harrison, C. (1963) 'Clergyman as Counsellor', *American Journal of Sociology*, pp. 234-43.
15. Piedmont, E. (1968) 'Referrals and Reciprocity: Psychiatrists, General Practitioners and Clergymen' *Journal of Health & Social Behaviour*, 9. pp. 29-41. The author found that clergymen only refer about a tenth of people coming to them with mental problems.
16. Kadushin, C. (1962) 'Social Distance between Client and Professional', *American Journal of Sociology*, 67, pp. 517-31.

17. Larson, R. (1968) 'The Clergyman's Role in the Therapeutic Process: Disagreement between Clergymen and Psychiatrists'. *Psychiatry*, 31, pp. 250-63.
18. Ibid, p. 262. The author found that psychiatrists made a greater claim to sole legitimacy in the therapeutic setting and that clergymen accepted this jurisdictional claim.
19. Cummings, E. op. cit. The author proposes that such working class clergymen are viewed as 'judgemental' by psychiatrists and therefore do not receive referrals. At the same time, clergymen may be aware of the agency's reluctance to deal with working class clients (in the American Setting).
20. Clausen, J. and Yarrow, M. (1955) 'Paths to the Mental Hospital'. *Journal of Social Issues*, pp. 25-32. The authors reported that 'clergy tended most often to be involved (by either husband or wife) in the early stages of a husband's symptomatic behaviour but seldom influenced the way the illness was dealt with'.
21. Cummings, E. op. cit.
22. Henderson, M. and Argyle, M. (1985) 'Source and Nature of Social Support given to Women at Divorce/Separation, *British Journal of Social Work*, 15, pp. 57-65.
23. Horowitz, A. (1978) 'Family, Kin and Friend Networks in Psychiatric Helpseeking', *Social Science and Medicine*, pp. 297-304.
24. Lowe, C. and Braaten, G. 'Differences in Religious Attitudes in Mental Illness', *Journal for the Scientific Study of Religion*, 5, pp. 435-45.
25. Sherman, M. and Sharman, I. (1934) 'Psychotic Symptoms and Social Backgrounds', in *The Problems of Mental Disorder*. Committee of Psychiatric Investigations, (National Research Council), Chapt. 18.
26. McDonald, C. and Luckett, J. (1983) 'Religious Affiliation and Psychiatric Diagnosis', *Journal for the Scientific Study of Religion*, 22, pp. 15-37. The authors analysed a sampe of 7,000 patients attending psychiatric clinic, acording to religion and diagnosis. Non-mainline Protestant is used to describe the evangelical churches. Main-line Protestant is used to include non-conformist and Presbyterian.
27. Murphy, H. and Vega, G. (1982) 'Schizophrenia and Religious Affiliation in Northern Ireland' *Psychological Medicine*, 12, pp. 595-605. Catholic schizophrenics predominated West of the Bann and resembled the situation in the West of Ireland; whilst, in the Protestant industrial east rates were low and similar to Englnd.
28. Murphy, H. (1975) 'Alcohol and Schizophrenia in the Irish: A Review', *Transcultural Psychiatric Research*, 12, pp. 116-39.
29. Dune, D. (1970) 'Psychiatric Problems in County Mayo', *Corridor Echo, Journal of St. Mary's Hospital*, Feb. 1970.
30. Scheper-Hughes, N. (1979) *Saints, Scholars and Schizophrenics*, Los Angeles.
31. Murphy, H. (1982) op. cit.
32. McDonald, C. and Luchett, J. (1983) op. cit.

7 The general practitioner

The general practitioner stands at the centre of the stage in the admission process to psychiatric hospital and, therefore, in the selection of what constitutes a psychiatric case. This is recognised in a World Health Organisation report that states 'the primary medical care team is the cornerstone of community psychiatry'.[1] The model presented in Chapter Three is constructed around the role of the general practitioner as the gatekeeper to the specialist psychiatric services.[2] In this model the G.P. identifies psychiatric cases amongst his patient population (Filter Two) and decides whether to treat such cases himself or refer them to the psychiatric out-patient clinic (Filter Three). The importance of the G.P. has been confirmed by research in Scotland where 78 per cent of new out-patients were referred by them[3] and in London where 75 per cent were so referred.[4]

However, such a model presumes a step by step progression through each filter. But in the present study only 18 per cent of admissions were filtered through community psychiatric services.[5] The majority of patients side-stepped or 'short-circuited' this filtering process, although this did not mean that the G.P. was not involved in these admissions.[6] Rather, the nature of his involvement varied with the parts played by other formal agencies (which will be discussed in the following chapters). The G.P.'s role varied from primary decision-maker to simply rubber-stamping the decisions of others. Furthermore, the G.P. does not act in a systematic and deliberate way to select psychiatric cases from his patient-load. More likely, he is besieged on all sides by prospective patients, relatives, and police and other agencies with demands for hospital admission. He then has to petition the hospital which may be in a similar position of siege. The G.P. is very much in the middle: on the one side faced with demands that 'something must be done'; on the other side being stonewalled by the hospital.

How family doctors deal with this situation, the strategies they develop, and the factors that influence their decision-making are discussed in the present chapter. Particularly important are attitudes of G.P.s, their work settings and the way they handle emergencies. The 'rules of thumb' and strategies developed by G.P.s to achieve hospitalisation are analysed and discussed.

Information was collected from G.P.s by conducting interviews based on open-ended questions aimed at encouraging the interviewee to discuss his style of work and attitude to psychiatric illness. Almost all G.P.s were seen who worked in the district in three Health Centres. In the biggest Centre G.P.s were interviewd individually and in the other two centres a group meeting was held. A single group practice operated from a private house and a representative G.P. was interviewed from this group. In total some eighteen family doctors were interviewed individually and in small groups.

A study of G.P.s in north-east Scotland has utilised similar semi-structured interviewing techniques.[7] Other researchers have administered structured questionnaires to groups of G.P.s; most well known of these is Michael Shepherd and his investigation of London family doctors.[8] Shepherd's study was also concerned with determining incidence of psychiatric illness and used case-finding techniques. Other studies have analysed referral letters sent by G.P.s to psychiatrists.[9] I did not have access to referral letters and in any case a significant numbers of patients had no written referral letters from their G.P. Where referral notes existed, they were often in the form of a prescription confirming details of a telephone conversation and had no case background. It was therefore necessary to rely on interviews with G.P.s.

Previous Research

Referral to a psychiatrist and admission to psychiatric hospital is not a straightforward process of assessment and referral. Rather, it has been described as a process that is 'devious and often arbitrary'.[10] Attempts to disentangle the crucial variables determining outcome in general practice have distinguished between social and demographic characteristics, and attitudinal factors. Researchers have found that demographic differences between practices are not sufficient to explain variations in referral rates.[11] Rather, other variables such as the mobility of patients in and out of G.P. practice;[12] the personal characteristics of the G.P.;[13] the G.P.'s feelings of stigma about mental hospitalisation;[14] and the G.P.'s experience of and attitude towards the local psychiatric service,[15] are of importance.

Research has found that the symptoms of psychiatric illness in general practice are often psychological symptoms of palpitations, headaches, tiredness, sleep disturance and tremors which may be exacerbated by stress.[16] Such stress factors occurr most often in women involved with problems of child-management, dependent relatives, housing difficulties and marital disharmoney, and are associated with the responsibilities of the female role.[17] Patients who are more likely to have their symptoms detected are female, middle-aged, separated, divorced or widowed, and unemployed and those seen most frequently at the surgery.[18]

Research has principally been concerned with case-identification and estimates of psychiatric morbidity. Such work assumes that deciding what constitutes psychiatric illness is not a problem. By such screening techniques as the General Health Questionnaire and Present State Examination, psychiatric cases are defined across time and space. Earlier theoretical discussion in Chapter Three has outlined the weaknesses inherent in such a position. However, the concern of the present investigation is not with the measurement of prevalence or with methods of case identification or symptomatology but with the intangibles of decision-making, the idiosyncracies that determine actions, and the informal codes of conduct.

Work Settings and Philosophies

The district is made up of three distinct geographical entitities: Area A. - public housing; Area B. - private housing; and Area C. - rural. Each geographical area is served by its own Health Centre. Attitudinal factors are likely to be influenced by and mediated through the characteristics of the work setting and the catchment areas. G.P.s, like other occupational groups, need to make sense of their work activities by the development of 'work philosophies'. The characteristics and attitudes of each catchment area will be discussed in turn.

Area A. contains considerable urban deprivation and makes high demands on the local Health Centre. City practices, where some patients make greater demands on doctors, also make more psychiatric referrals than rural practices.[19] A moralistic stance or a sociological explanation were the main attitudinal consequences. Although more recently trained, taught more psychiatry and required to work in psychiatric settings in their training, younger doctors, with less experience, were more moralistic and judgemental than older doctors. Older doctors with greater experience have been found to make more psychiatric referrals. This may be explained by their lack of interest in treating psychiatric cases or by the high demands on their time.[20]

Some doctors were critical of patients with psychiatric problems and described them as ignorant and said that they 'couldn't be pleased'. That such views were expressed by younger doctors suggests the inclusion of theories of social causation of mental illness in their training has made little impression. Interestingly, one doctor occupied a half-way position in which the need for health education was emphasised without much hope of it achieving results. This doctor seemed to have a disproportionate number of 'difficult patients' who made greater demands for tranquillisers and psychiatric hospitalisation. Because this doctor was one of the youngest in the practice, she may well have been obliged to take on the least desirable patients. On the other hand, the patients themselves may have sought her out in the hope of achieving their demands.

Older and more experienced doctors were more likely to use sociological explanations of psychiatric breakdown; perhaps evidence of a more benign and sympathetic attitude towards their patients. For example, they searched for environmental stresses such as poverty as explanations for depression. One doctor found it hard to understand and sympathise with materially well-off middle class patients who complained of depression. In general terms, this group saw medicine as taking over from the church and meeting similar needs. The heavy demands on medical services made by people living in a deprived area had brought about a more pragmatic, and less scientific approach. It is in this way that the characteristics of the catchment area influence G.P.s' attitudes. Something similar will be described for other 'gatekeepers'.

The doctors working in Area B. also used a sociological explanation of the effects of a pocket of deprivation in an otherwise relatively well-off area of private housing. The high rate of overdosing reported from this deprived spot was explained by the lack of social cohesion and family support with the area being described as a 'social engineering disaster'. Such explanations serve to normalise behaviour and offer a rationale for avoiding medical diagnosis and hospital admission. Area B. doctors may have operated as more effective gatekeepers because they knew all their present psychiatric cases and reckoned on only one new case a year. Because of the lower level of demand doctors were better acquainted with patients' circumstances and were less pressed by emergencies. As a result a more formal model of mental illness operated in which the distinction between 'real' mental illness and environmentally produced stress related behaviour could be maintained.

Finally, Area C. is a rural area where G.P.s held more traditional attitudes to mental illness. One G.P. stated a marked reluctance to request psychiatrist domiciliaries for fear that 'if the people see the psychiatrist, they might be able to get round him and get into hospital'. On the other hand, there was some evidence of earlier referral to the psychiatric services which may have reflected lower levels of tolerance of unusual behaviour. Another factor was the greater distance to the nearest casualty unit which encouraged earlier referral of the potentially suicidal. Individual doctors maintained their own theoretical bias and there were differences of opinion amongst G.P.s in their attitude towards psychiatric disposal. In this setting, it was the older doctors who appeared more rigid and uncompromising.

Attitudes to Psychiatry and the Psychiatric Services

Previous research in England and Ireland has emphasised the crucial importance of attitudes in determining outcome of psychiatric referral in general practice. In his London study, Shepherd found that the two most frequent reasons for not referring were the stigma of mental illness and the attitude to the local psychiatric service.[21] When this study was replicated in Ireland, it was found that Irish doctors were even more aware of the associated stigma attached to psychiatric referral than their English counterparts.[22] The present study showed evidence of a similar attitude in Northern Ireland.

In some cases the G.P. was more concerned than patients about the stigma attached to mental hospitalisation. That this indicated an underlying negative attitude towards mental illness cannot be stated. Doctors were concerned about the ways in which mental hospitalisation may affect employment and life insurance for their patients. There was a tendency for G.P.s to ignore disruptive behaviour and avoid labelling which indicated that G.P.s shared public attitudes of denial of mental illness. One doctor made a comparison between how he would like to be treated and what he was being asked to do and acting accordingly. Doctors accept family pressure to arrange hospital admission because this means that responsibility for such a decision is shared.

To hospitalise an unwilling patient, the family doctor may have to use his legal authority. For some doctors using compulsory powers of detention was an unpleasant task. For example, one doctor stated 'a thing not to be done lightly and only when you have had to go a long way down that line of disturbed behaviour'. The use of power is disguised in the normal doctor-patient relationship and stems from the accepted authority and expertise vested in the doctor's position. Doctors generally continue to believe in an idealised version of doctor/patient interaction in which they serve patients and act in their interest to cure their ills. Such occupational values rest uneasy with the possession of legal powers of compulsion. One G.P. admitted that working class patients were easier to deal with because they were less aware of their rights and legal procedure. In contrast, middle class patients appeared to be treated warily, particularly if they arrived at the surgery armed with legal documents as in one case reported!

The way in which the Health Service is structured gives general practitioners no direct right of access to hospital beds and this is a general grievance for them. Obtaining a hospital bed requires negotiation with a hospital doctor who can be a house officer, the junior of the G.P. Over the period of the study there was only one occasion when a hospital doctor other than a consultant directly opposed a family doctor. This occurred when a G.P. used the police to send an intoxicated person to the hospital in the middle of the night without any prior negotiation. The duty doctor challenged the G.P. and a furious row ensued in which the latter emphasised his seniority.

In general, G.P. and consultant are mutually dependent and respect the boundaries of their responsibiliies. The hospital consultant is dependent on the G.P. for patients and the G.P. dependent on the consultant for hospital beds. The consultant encourages this relationship in order to influence the G.P. in his selection of patients for psychiatric referral. The presentation of the results of this study to a group of hospital consultants provoked some disappointment that their efforts to improve liason and understanding had not produced better results.

The opinion of G.P.s about the local psychiatric service and their past experience of it has been shown to be a crucial factor in determining referral. One research study found that 29 per cent of G.P.s in London gave previous delay in getting a psychiatric appointment as a reason for non-referral,[23] although there was less dissatisfaction with the psychiatric services reported in Ireland.[24] In the present study attitudes varied with the level of demand. Area B. doctors working in a suburban area with manageable workloads had a benign attitude to the local psychiatric service and informal contacts with the psychiatrists. The working distinction emphasised by the local psychiatrist between those with 'genuine' mental illness who could be helped, and others with 'problems of living' who should not be labelled mentally ill, was accepted and workable by local doctors. Indeed, local G.P.s voiced their criticism of hospital doctors as 'hooked on diagnosis' and saw such 'living' problems as normal reactions to stress. Strains were more evident in the case of fringe groups of both undesirable and troublesome patients whose disposal was a matter for negotiation with hospital and police, neither of which wished to be involved.

Area B. doctors were not critical of the local psychiatric service and described the delay in outpatient appointments as 'not too bad'. This delay was itself seen as useful in allowing the doctor time to assess properly the situation. Domiciliary visits by the psychiatrist to the patient's home were also seen as useful 'in taking the heat out of the situation'. It was difficult to form an overall impression of the use of such tactics but such visits were made in situations of 'semi-crisis', perhaps as a less stigmatising method of contact with the psychiatric services for the better-off.

The harder-worked G.P.s of Area A, an area of high social deprivation, were more critical. One described his efforts to admit a patient to hospital as 'it being easier to get into heaven!'. Other aspects of the service that were also criticised included the out-patient clinic which involved delays that meant 'something acute had passed by the time of the appointment', and domiciliaries were not quick enough to deal with emergencies. Clearly, where G.P.s experienced heavy demands on their services strains in their relationship with the local psychiatric service were more evident. Psychiatrists may have felt some collegiate solidarity with their medical colleagues, but their priority was the defence of their territorial domain against the demands of 'undesirable' patients.

Where attitude to the local psychiatric service was a crucial factor in determining referral, Shepherd described such practice as 'contingency doctoring'. He found that a crucial test of the effectiveness of the local psychiatric service for family doctors was its response to the 'sociomedical problems of old age'. In the present study, it was found that G.P.s were preoccupied with the problems of finding hospital treatment for elderly patients. Its significance was also underlined by the fact that consultants themselves intervened in the assessment of such referrals. G.P.s were, in general, critical of the lack of response from the hospital and consultants were seen as being only concerned with 'not getting their beds blocked'.

At the time of study, a new psycho-geriatric unit to be built at the hospital was still at the planning stage and the mushrooming of private residential care had not yet occurred. Consequently, there were very few facilities to look after an increasingly elderly population. Social Services residential homes had waiting lists of at least a year long and long-stay hospital wards rarely had an empty bed.

With the elderly, G.P.s were particularly open to pressure from relatives, neighbours, social workers and police, and were particularly aggrieved about a perceived lack of response from the local psychiatric service. G.Ps saw domicilary visits as a way of involving the psychiatrist in a situation requiring him to face up to the demands from everybody that 'something must be done'. In one case, an alternative response was to use personal contacts with doctors outside the catchment area to gain a hospital bed.

The Psychiatric Emergency

The preceding chapter has described the way in which families only seek psychiatric hospitalisation as a last resort. Such points of breakdown often appear as psychiatric emergencies, in which either some item of outrageous or unacceptable behaviour, or the total accumulation of various behaviours mean that family tolerance has been breached and immediate removal of the offender is demanded. It is in such situations that the G.P. is required to operate.

Both Rawnsley and Loudon in South Wales[25] and Robertson in Western Scotland[26] found that pressure from relatives was an important influence in bringing about psychiatric referral. There was ample evidence in the present study of the influence of relatives and other agencies, although this was partly a two-way process. Relatives were the single largest group initiating contact with G.P. although it was also possible for a G.P. to initiate contact with relatives in order to substantiate a patient's account. G.P.s reported being faced with a chorus of people demanding action which effectively meant removal of the offender. Once the G.P. bowed to such pressure, the question effectively became one of destination or disposal. G.P.s predictably felt angry and frustrated when they were stonewalled by the local psychiatric service.

In certain circumstances, delay in psychiatric assessment was viewed as useful as a means 'to keep the case under tabs for three or four days'. However, often the G.P. is required to make an immediate response when, because he is the duty doctor at night or weekend, he is unfamiliar with the case. In such situations of uncertainty, most professionals err on the side of caution. Although the family doctor may have left instructions as to how to handle the case, the main priority in the middle of the night is finding a satisfactory solution which, more often or not, is removal.

Relationships with other professional groups are another source of pressure for the hard-pressed G.P. The management of emergency situations often involves the police and G.P.s enlisting their help to deal with violence. It was apparent that relationships between G.P.s and police were mutually beneficial on a practical level. G.P.s appreciated police assistance and protection in handling threatening situations. The police, in their turn, relied on the doctor to deal with incomprehensible and bizarre behaviour.This relationship could become strained and there was some grumbling about the police being over eager to medicalise behaviour in order to 'get Joe out of the barracks'. This was evident in one comment made by a G.P. that 'it was the Sergeant who made the diagnosis'.

Outcome is determined by the negotiation between professional groups according to their relative bargaining power. It is also influenced by the extent to which occupational groups are dependent on each other, and the alternative sources of help, places of disposal and strategies of intervention which are available to them.

The Selling of Referral

Given the stigma attached to being labelled mentally ill, doctors may have a problem arranging psychiatric help for patients. As they do not like using their statutory powers of formal admission G.P.s must try to persuade patients that they need help. Circumlocution plays an important part in such persuasion. Previous research has found that over a third of patients referred to a psychiatric out-patient clinic for the first time were not aware that they were to see a psychiatrist. Half of them were distressed to discover this fact, and two-thirds felt that their G.P. had not told them anything about what to expect.[27]

What emerged from G.P. interviews was that the nature of psychiatric referral tended to be blurred and couched in such phrases as 'needing to see a specialist' or 'getting a second opinion'. Statements such as 'done all I can', 'run out of ideas', and 'can't do anything more' described the G.P.'s inability to cure and paved the way for suggesting some expert help. Another strategy was to emphasise the fact that such specialists have more time and expertise, although in practice it seems that psychiatric consultations are also becoming increasingly hurried. The fact that G.P.s sometimes failed to mention to the patient that they were referring them to a psychiatrist indicates their own discomfort with psychiatry, a fact that G.P.s were only too ready to admit. Considerable effort in health education has been directed to promoting the view that mental illness is the same as physical illness. G.P.s put forward similar ideas in persuading patients to accept psychiatric referral. Where such methods were ineffective doctors were prepared to use their powers of compulsion, although the threat of compulsion was sometimes sufficient to achieve hospitalisation.

Rules of Thumb

'Rules of thumb' provide the basis on which family doctors judge behaviour in their daily work. Research on G.P.s and mental illness has concentrated on aspects of case identification and estimates of size and magnitude. Methods used have been of the questionnaire type which involve G.P.s reporting on their own behaviour and beliefs. Such reporting is open to distortion as the respondent seeks to present himself in the best possible light. One method of research that has avoided this problem is the analysis of G.P. referral letters requesting psychiatric hospital admission. A West of Scotland study found that few practitioners referred patients on the basis of positive diagnostic appraisal. Rather they tended to stress abnormalities of conduct, the existence of social problems or inappropiate responses to medical treatment as reasons for referral.[28]

My own findings confirm that doctors emphasised the ensuing disruptive or concern-provoking behaviour as a reason for hospitalisation. The only diagnosis regularly referred to was depression which may have been a reflection of the fact that there had been a number of recent suicides. All G.P.s stated they would seek admission for patients who were suicidal although it was not immediately clear how the seriousness of a suicidal threat was measured. It was recognised that old rules of thumb like 'if they threatened suicide, they won't do it' could not be relied upon. G.P.s were clearly concerned to protect themselves from any accusation that they had failed to act to prevent suicide. The high referral rate for those expressing suicidal intent was also reported in the Scottish study where 70 per cent of G.P.s said they would not attempt to treat suicidal or severely depressed patients[29].

The Scottish study also found the highest rate of referral for psychotic patients; 90 per cent of G.P.s saying that they would always refer them.[30] Although hallucinations and delusions were given as grounds for referral by G.P.s in the present study, aggression or the threat of violence which sometimes, although not necessarily, accompanies psychotic behaviour was mentioned more often. Rather than the diagnosing of psychotic behaviour, the primary concern was the management and containment of anti-social behaviour. Threatening parents, throwing the dinner across the room, breaking windows and throwing ornaments were some examples of legitimate grounds for referral as long as these behaviours were accompanied by other signs of disturbance. One recognised rule of thumb for G.P.s was to check there were no charges pending in cases of aggressive behaviour to avoid hospital being used as 'a bolt hole instead of litigation'.

The G.P. builds up a composite picture of an individual from reports of changes in behaviour and changes in personality in different arenas of activity, and, on this basis, decides if hospitalisation is required. Much of such information comes from relatives and other parties who themselves have a vested interest in the outcome of the doctor's decision. It is in such situations that the G.P. is open to pressure from relatives.

Accumulated beliefs have been outlined in a previous section and they are clearly a vital determinant in decision-making. There are also variables of a more occupational nature which relate directly to the nature of the work. For instance, there was a general prediliction for activity: having been called out to a case in the middle of the night, it was likely that the G.P. would act if only to ensure that he would not be called out again. Similarly compulsory powers are used to ensure that the person will go to hospital and not be a source of further referral. In the words of one G.P., 'having gone to the trouble of getting him a bed, he's got to stay if he's going to get any treatment'.

Frequency of contact is an important variable in deciding psychiatric referral. One doctor suggested that after seeing a patient five or six times he would consider psychiatric referral. Not simply frequency of contact but also length of time without improvement are crucial. G.Ps have a range of medication available and regularly use such types as anti-depressants. However, it became clear that where the major tranquillisers were needed because of the potential for side-effects. G.P.s would most refer such patients to the psychiatric services.

Time is crucial for the family doctor and one researcher has viewed the request for psychiatric referral by the G.P. as a request for relief from his own stress.[31] The G.P. is in the front line of the medical services and has to face a daily demand for actions which he sometimes cannot meet. Having experienced an unsympathetic response to his admission enquiry, the G.P. may well feel that the hospital doctor does not appreciate the level of pressure he is facing.

G.P.s are asked to make judgements of social behaviour and social situations when they make decisons about psychiatric referral. In making such judgements they will be influenced by a whole range of emotions, experiences and values. However, when a patient keeps returning to the surgery with the same litany of complaints, the G.P. may well refer him out of desperation. By such idiosyncracies and fortuitous events, definitions of mentally ill behaviour are made. The verification of the definition of behaviour as mentally ill is made by the psychiatric services. Whether this confirmation is forthcoming is a matter of negotiation between the respective 'gate-keeping' agencies.

A Prospective Model

Diagram One attempts to encapsulate the position of the G.P. as gatekeeper, determining outcome and the alternatives to hospital. It is important to emphasise that G.P.s not only persuade reluctant patients but also prevent the admission of those whom they are not prepared to endorse as sick. A case example might best bring alive the social contingencies involved and the institutional responses to them.

> A young man caused a rumpus at the Health Centre when he felt he had been left waiting too long, and threatened to harm himself. The police were called to remove him. However, when this man threatened suicide in his police cell the police contacted his family doctor. His G.P. refused to have anything to do with him and struck him off the practice register. The police turned to the police doctor for ratification of their medicalisation of his behaviour. The man was believed a risk, his bootlaces had been removed and the police wanted him transferred to hospital. The police doctor was expected 'to get him away'. However, the hospital were adamant in their refusal to admit him. At the same time, the police doctor would not let him be released because, in his own words, 'if he killed himself who would be responsible . . . me!'. The police doctor made him a compulsory patient to ensure his admission to hospital and sent him up to the hospital in an ambulance. However, the hospital stood firm in their refusal on instruction from the consultant. In the event, the ambulance was turned away and left to go elsewhere and the individual was not admitted.

In this case, the behaviour that needed to be responded to was the threat of self-harm. The strategy adopted by his G.P. was to strike the patient off the panel and thereby abdicate responsibility for him. In this way the G.P. was able to counteract what he saw as deliberate manipulation by the patient to be admitted to hospital. The hospital adopted a similar stance and refused involvement. The police were concerned to remove the man from the station in a satisfactory disposal which transferred their responsibility. This 'social tidying-up' was the task of the police doctor (a G.P. colleague from the same Health Centre) who was critical of his colleague's refusal to be involved. Once the man had been sent to the hospital, responsibility for him was regarded as transferred.

Such are the professional and institutional responses in situations of labelling which are contested. For the most part, G.P.s' decisions are accepted and admission follows. This case is useful in demonstrating the strategies available and the negotiation between gatekeepers. The G.P. has an armoury of responses to the psychiatric case ranging from persuasion, seduction, to threats and compulsory hospitalisation. Other alternatives are to normalise behaviour (why not go away on holiday?); prevarication (built-in to the system by the delay in out-patient appointments and domiciliaries); referral to other agencies; and disengagement (striking off the panel). In response, the psychiatric service can utilise various strategies in 'suspicious' cases from lengthy waiting-lists, 'no beds available', to 'blacklisting'. The G.P., in turn, can engage the hospital by strategies such as formal commitment. Finally, the pre-patient and his complainants can adopt threatening tactics: to dump a relative; to self-harm and to hold the G.P. responsible. These are the realities of hospital admission; the interaction the social process of psychiatric hospitalisation.

Diagram One; The Referral Process

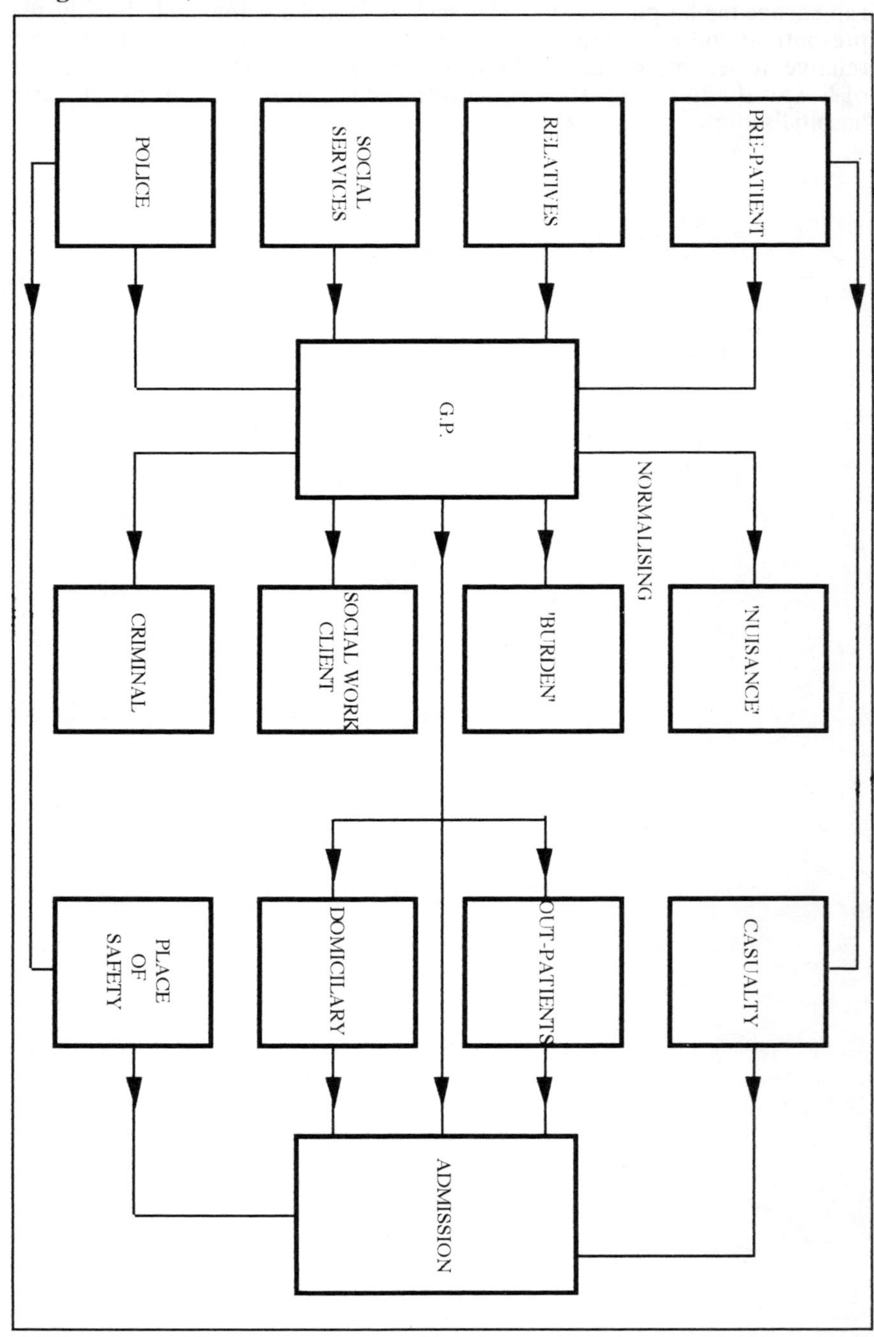

Notes

1. Report of Working Group, (1973) *Psychiatry and Primary Medical Care*, Copenhagen WHO.
2. Goldberg, D. and Huxley, P. (1980) *Mental Illness in the Community*, London.
3. Robertson, N. (1979) 'Variations in Referral Pattern to the Psychiatric Services by General Practitioners', *Psychological Medicine*, 9, pp. 355-64.
4. Taylor, L. and Chave, S. (1964) *Mental Health and the Environment*, London.
5. Mezey, A. and Evans, E. (1971) 'Psychiatric In-patients and Out-Patients in a London Borough', *British Journal of Psychiatry*, 118, pp. 609-16. This study found that 30 per cent of admissions were filtered through community psychiatric services.
6. Ibid. A figure of 45 per cent was reported for this group in this study.
7. Robertson, N. (1979) op. cit.
8. Shepherd, M., Cooper, B., Brown, A. and Kalton, G. (1966) *Psychiatric Illness in General Practice*, London.
9. Mowbray, R., Blair, W., Jubb. L. and Clarke, A. (1961) 'The General Practitioners Attitude to Psychiatry', *Scottish Medical Journal*, pp. 314-21.
10. Kessel, N. (1963) 'Who Ought to see a Psychiatrist', pp. 1092-5. 18th May 1963.
11. Rawnsley, K. and Loudon, J. (1962) 'Factors Influencing the Referral of Patients to Psychiatrists by General Practitioners', *British Journal of Preventative Social Medicine*. 16, pp. 174-82.
12. Shepherd, M. et al (1966) op. cit.
13. Mowbray, R. et al. (1961) op. cit.
14. Fahey, T., O'Rourke, A. and Wilson-Davis, K. 'The Irish Family Doctor and Psychiatry', *Journal of the Irish Medical Association*, 67, December 7, 1974, pp. 616-24.
15. Taylor, L. and Chave, S. (1964) op. cit.
16. Goldberg, D. and Huxley, P. (1980) op. cit.
17. Shepherd, M. et al. (1966) op. cit.

18. Marks, J., Goldberg, D. and Hillier, V. (1979) 'Determinants of the Ability of G.P.s to detect Psychiatric Illness', *Psychological Medicine*, 9, pp. 357-73.
19. Robertson, N. (1979) op. cit.
20. Mowbray, R. et al (1961) op. cit.
21. Shepherd, M. (1966) op. cit.
22. Fahey, T. et al (1974) op. cit.
23. Shepherd, M. (1966) op. cit. 40% of English doctors gave delay in psychiatric appointments as a reason for non-referral.
24. Fahey, T. et al (1974) op. cit. Only 9% of Irish doctors gave delay in appointment as a reason for non-referral.
25. Rawnsley, K. and Loudon, J. (1962) op. cit.
26. Robertson, N. (1979) op. cit.
27. Skuse, D. (1975) 'Attitudes to the Psychiatric Outpatient Clinic' *British Medical Journal*, 23 August 1975, pp. 469-71.
28. Mowbray, R. et al (1961) op. cit.
29. Robertson, N. (1979) op. cit.
30. Ibid.
31. Anderson, D. (1972) 'Working with the Family Doctor: A Programme for Mental Health', *British Medical Journal*, 4, pp. 781-4.

8 The police

Compulsory Hospitalisation

The operation of social control in the labelling of mental illness is most obviously seen in the practice of compulsory admission. Sociologists have taken a particular interest in its application and their research has been used as evidence to support the labelling perspective.[1] However, confining interest only to compulsory hospitalisation is restrictive as the distinction between voluntary (informal) and involuntary (formal) admission is rather arbitrary. For instance, the fact that compulsory powers exist can be used as a sanction to persuade a reluctant patient to enter hospital 'voluntarily'. Informal admission may mean only that a patient has been successfully threatened with formal admission. Similarly, in hospital, a reluctant voluntary patient can be prevailed upon to stay and agree to treatment by the threat of compulsory detention. The level of compulsory admission is, therefore, only an indicator of the extent to which authorities have resorted to legal powers to detain people in hospital. It does not give an accurate indication of the extent to which coercive methods are used to bring people into hospital.

As a corollary, it is important to state that the agencies of social control - in this case the police, social services and psychiatric services - operate not only in a coercive way but also in a conciliatory and supportive manner. The present study found that 20 per cent of admissions were involuntary which is somewhat higher level than recent English figures,[2] and compares with the English situation in the 1960's.[3] However, it has been found that there is considerable variation in the use of compulsory hospitalisation over time and between regions.[4] This would seem to reflect local practices and individual policies, and Mental Welfare Officers, prior to 1961, have been found to be strongly influenced by local authority policy in their actions.[5] It seems that labelling activity by the police in borderline areas such as drug and alcohol addiction establishes local boundaries for whether such activity is interpreted as criminal or psychiatric.[6] Local practices of law enforcement in these quasi-legal decisions are complementary between the police and pyschiatric services so that lower involvement of the police in a particular area of deviance is balanced by a higher concern of psychiatrists.[7]

Compulsory admission has been a preoccupation of sociologists concerned to justify the labelling perspective. The fact that the lower social classes are much more likely to be admitted compulsorily[8] has been used by proponents and critics of the labelling perspective.[9] The working class's lack of power, lack of enlightenment about the medical model, fatalistic attitude towards 'troubles', and fear of being incarcerated have all been cited as explanations for their high rates of compulsory admission.[10] Psychiatric emergencies involving compulsory admission have been described as reflecting 'disruptive and flamboyant behaviour (which is) more likely to happen in the lower social classes'.[11]

Studies of police activity have found that it is not low social class but lack of accessibility to other community resources that determines resort to the police for help.[12] In the present study, the social class breakdown of formal admissions reflects the social class breakdown of the sample as a whole which is overwhelmingly working class (See Appendix Three). The living arrangements of those admitted compulsorily is also similar to the whole of the sample and there is not a disproportionate number of people living alone, as might have been expected.[13] The behaviour exhibited by those formally admitted is also representative of the sample as a whole. The main difference is that formal agencies, predictably, are more often involved in compulsory admissions than voluntary ones. It is important to emphasise that involvement of law officers does not necesarily mean formal admission. The unique feature of the police as labellers will be outlined, with illustration from the present study and from my informal conversation with the police about their involvement in referral to psychiatric hospital. This is followed by an elaboration of the conventional wisdom which guides their intervention.

Police Activity

The police, like all members of society, engage with the world through an assemblage of background expectations and norms: what Cicourel calls 'a sense of social structure'.[14] It is the way in which the police come to 'read' the social environment and convert displays of the everyday world into recognisable situations in which they can act in certain predetermined ways, that is of interest. The question is one of how the police come to use the label of mental illness in their occupational activity. In this task, they do not have a predetermined view of mental illness in their official ideology, and the legislation which they are required to enforce does not contain practical guidelines as to how law enforcement should occur.[15]

The policeman has a unique function as a decisive, authority figure who can be called upon to resolve issues of social control. In moments of personal and family crisis it has been found that the public turns first to the police as figures of authority.[16] The police view it as a basic responsibility to respond to all calls, firstly, because of their occupational value 'to serve the public', and, secondly, because there is a complaints procedure to which the public can resort if dissatisfied. There are two main ways in which the police cope with this all-embracing responsibility; they can seek to normalise behaviour and they can refer it elsewhere.

Normalisation

The police bring to their daily work a set of values and beliefs that they are likely to share with the general public. Predictably, it has been found that the police avail themselves of various forms of denial when confronted with behaviour regarded as mentally ill.[17] A reluctance to label may be explained by a greater tolerance of deviant behaviour brought about by frequent demands upon them to isolate and control people who are disrupting the social order and who are unwilling to change their behaviour. For instance, the particular setting of an inner-city area is likely to necessitate frequent contact with transient people behaving in odd ways.[18]

Bittner noted that the police dealt with such behaviours by 'psychiatric first-aid'. The police responded in a normal police way to bizarre complaints which were accepted at face value but then went away and did nothing about them.[19] Whether labelling takes place depends in part on whether the person has the previously ascribed status of psychiatric patient. Mendel found previous hospitalisation was a significant variable for hospital doctors in determining readmission.[20] Previous history of hospital admission is likely to facilitate readmision and make hospitalisation a feasible alternative.

The police may act on the advice of the psychiatric services in order to apprehend a named individual and convey to hospital. Transport of detained individuals to hospital is one of the duties of the police and is outlined in their procedural manual. In responding to 999 calls, the police may judge situations as requiring medical help and provide transport (or arrange an ambulance) for individuals to the casualty units of the general hospitals. The disposal of such cases then becomes the responsibility of the hospital doctor. For example, following an overdose or inflicted self-harm, disposal is quite straightforward. Medical treatment is required and the police will facilitate it. The following case illustrates the process.

> 'A' is an elderly lady who lives alone and had telephoned the police several times a day over a long period to complain about her flat being under surveillamce and her life being in danger. She reported that her downstairs neighbour had been trying to poison her with fumes and had contaminated her tap water. The police responded by calling on her frequently, listening to her complaints and then going away and doing nothing about them. This situation continued until 'A' threw water on the stairs of her elderly neighbour's. The water froze which made the stairs very dangerous. When her neighbour complained to social services, they, in turn, arranged with the police for a police doctor to call. Admission was duly arranged. On two subsequent occasions, following 'A's return home to attend the Day Hospital, she stopped attending and disappeared from her flat. On each occasion the police were contacted to find her and return her to hospital.

This case is a good example of 'psychiatric first-aid'. Only when 'A'. endangers a neighbour who is a social services client is her behaviour drawn to the attention of another formal agency. This agency is then prepared to act because of the risk to their own client. However, following discharge and 'A's disappearance, the function of the police changes to that of locating a missing psychiatric patient and it is no longer possible for them to ignore her behaviour. In general, police involvement in psychiatric hospitalisation centres around destructive behaviour (attacks against persons and property), confusion (wandering), creating a social nuisance and suicidal behaviour.[21]

Passing Responsibility

The extent to which the police are the real decision-makers is debatable. They decide whether the problem is a police one or not and, if not, who is the appropriate agency to deal with it. In general terms, the police are reluctant to become involved unless behaviour is really bizarre, in which case the police doctor makes a decision about disposal. The priority for the police is 'keeping the peace'.[22] They are, therefore, concerned to find a solution for the problems brought to their attention. It is in this sense that the police are described as 'the secret social service'.[23] For example, one of the ways that the police pass on problem-solving responsibility to social services in the case of homeless (vagrant) people is to insist that they are unable to keep someone in the police station overnight without charging them.

There are certain instances when the police will be very keen to maintain a criminal perspective on behaviour, and this may bring them into conflict with psychiatrists. This is particularly true in the area of child sexual abuse, which may reflect the present police and public sensitivity to this issue. Psychiatrists are also anxious to ensure that their patient is not seeking to decriminalise impending court appearances by hospitalisation. Folk-lore has it that hospital staff in the early seventies were wary about people seeking hospitalisation as a refuge from illegal organisations. By such activities people re-create social institutions and structures to meet their own needs.

The ways in which the police act as labellers of mental illness is best described by example. In the present study it was found that the police acted in three types of situation: where an overt social nuisance, which could not be ignored, had been committed; where aggression had taken place within the family and the police had been called to intercede; and where the police performed a 'service' role for those in distress by linking them with a source of help. Each of these situations will be examined in turn.

Social Nuisance

Bittner describes police intervenion in situations involving serious disorentation, when someone 'by acting incongruously, creates a nuisance in a public place'.[26] This involves consideration of the visibility of deviance when the act of deviance draws attention to itself. This may take the form of loss of control over appearance, such as nudity. Bittner also emphasises the efforts that policemen make to return a person to a place of shelter if expediently possible. The following case illustrates some of these factors in operation.

> 'X's behaviour is highly tolerated by her family with whom she lives; effectively she is in the position of someone who lives alone and to whom attention is only drawn when she infringes social norms in a public place. This occurred when she shouted abuse outside a neighbour's house in the middle of the night and threw a brick through his window. Her behaviour conformed to the public stereotype of madness and the police acted on their own authority to bring her directly to hospital. This behaviour was clearly so unambiguous that the police were prepared to act immediately and their labelling was subsequently substantiated by her previous psychiatric history.

The police acted independently because of the unambiguous nature of the behaviour, the unsociable hour of the emergency, and the demands from the injured party. Clearly the police hold established ideas about what constitutes behaviour that cannot be ignored and requires defining as mentally ill, but their limits of tolerance of disturbed behaviour will be influenced by the amount of pressure from other parties. This, in turn, is also determined by the degree of perceived danger. In this case, not only was there someone demanding that something be done but this complainant also perceived himself and his family to be in danger.

In another case, a man with previous hospital admissions threw his television out of his tenth floor flat. The police were called and this man's failure to give a rational explanation and his previously ascribed patient status made hospitalisation an appropriate solution. A final example of police referral is provided by a woman who phoned the police staion to accuse them of watching her home and claimed to them that 'she was going to take over Ulster's divisions and Paisley would stand down'.

Behaviour labelled by the police as mentally ill is bizarre, and occurs in public. It involves visible acts of deviance and hospitalisation often requires the use of coercive methods. How far the police are prepared to tolerate behaviour is influenced by the demands from others for them to do something. Most commonly in cases of domestic violence, what is being demanded is the removal of the identified perpetrator.

Family Demands

The police are reluctant to intervene in situations which they perceive as family quarrels except or until there is 'extreme husband-wife conflict'.[27] The crucial determinant is the degree of danger or 'risk' as judged by the police who will seek to negotiate the situation from its dangerous phase to one of relative safety and normality. They will use their everyday police methods of 'keeping the peace' to achieve this aim. The police bring to the management of all situations the same 'on the job' skills and justifications for the way in which they act. In most cases of family violence the level of risk is less clearly defined, and the responsibility for the violence may be viewed as one shared by all the family. The police have a widely held occupational value of avoiding becoming involved in situations of 'domestic violence' a view they justify in the phrase 'it is a family affair'.

Should the police be called to negotiate a family dispute, psychiatric hospitalisation is clearly a tempting solution. Not only does it satisfy the family by the removal of the offender, it also leaves the police without any further responsibility or tiresome paperwork. Whether the person has previously been a psychiatric patient is a crucial determinant; this was a feature of each of the three instances of police involvement in family disputes ending in hospital admission. Other determinants are the strength and resourcefulness of the complainant in pressurising agencies to act; the extent to which other agents have attempted to mediate and contain the situation; the degree of violence involved; and the number of complainants and the interests they represent. Each of these factors will be examined in turn with illustration.

> 'J' has been coming into hospital for the last five years since he was seventeen. Each admission followed some incident of family disruption; on this occasion J. had thrown the telephone through the window after an argument with his mother. However, in hospital, when J. broke a hospital window, he was discharged. When 'J' refused to leave, the police were called to remove him and brought him home. The police returned 'J' to hospital after his mother said she would not accept him at home. The hospital doctor refused to readmit him and 'J' jumped in a window to get back into hospital. His mother successfully involved an interest group to petition for 'J.'s continued hospitalisation. When he was again, subsequently, discharged, 'J.s homelessness and subsequent vagrancy were a responsibility that the police were most reluctant to assume and he continued to come into hospital from time to time.

This case demonstrates the extent to which the police resisted a reinterpretation of behaviour which the hospital sought to impose. Clearly for the police, 'mentally ill' was a master status for 'J'. The degree to which police intervention represented 'the most marked discontinuities' in dealing with the patient's illness,[25] is also illustrated by the following case.

> Of three elderly sisters who lived together, 'B' was viewed by the other two as demanding, dominating and hard to please. They described her as 'boisterous and quarrelsome' for the previous two months and had tried to pacify her by indulging her, at the same time as calling a doctor who prescribed her sedation. However, soon after 'B' threw an ornament across the room and banged her

sister's head against the wall. A neighbour was called in to help and was also hit. He telephoned the police who called and admonished the offender. It was established she had previously been a hospital patient and a doctor arranged admission. In hospital, the need for her admission was viewed with some scepticism until the frailty of her sisters was revealed.

In this case, the involvement of a neighbour was important in mobilising additional support for removal; the other significant factor was that unsuccessful efforts had already been made to contain the situation prior to admission. From the G.P.'s point of view the police involvement reinforced the need for a more drastic solution. From the police's point of view, the G.P.'s previous involvement indicated a medical solution. Such is the way hospital admissions are negotiated and respective roles reaffirmed.

The police's willingness to act as negotiators in petitioning for hospital admission is confirmed by the final case in this category in which the police removed a drunk son from his mother's house at the request of a neighbour following the son's aggression to his mother. He was then kept in a cell overnight before being taken to hospital as a detained patient.

'Social Service'

The police may sometimes link people in distress with perceived sources of help. All three cases of this type involve young women of varying degrees of independence who had variously drawn atention to themselves. It may be that they conformed to a stereotype of latter-day 'damsels in distress', and hospitalisation may be viewed as a chivalrous response.

Two of these cases were very similar; both involved teenage girls who had fought with their parents and when drunk, away from home, had cut their wrists. One girl claimed she had been on her way to the police station in the expectation of finding a woman police constable to talk to. The police contacted her parents who sought advice from her doctor and he suggested hospital admission. In the second case, a friend of the distressed young woman made a 999 call and she was brought to the station. The police called a doctor who suggested coming into hospital for a rest to which the young woman agreed. In both cases, the police acted as facilitator to mobilise resources. As the self inflicted injuries were not serious enough to require casualty attention, the police involved the G.P.

In the third example a young woman was caught shoplifting but her medical condition was unclear. Both the shop manager and the police felt she was 'in a dazed state' and a doctor was called to the police station. According to the young woman, the doctor put it to her that the police had suggested sending her to hospital. This was duly arranged. In this case, police were able to decriminalise an act by medicalisation.

Research suggests that such social aspects of police work have a low priority in police culture which values 'rare moments of excitement and unambiguity'.[26] Policemen would rather see themselves solving difficult crimes, catching dangerous criminals and upholding public safety. This view requires modification; in the first place it is drawn from the American police and cannot necessarily be applied to suburban Northern Ireland where there are important cultural differences. In the second place, even if such an occupational ideology exists, the reality of the policeman 'on the beat' is one of 'keeping the peace'. In this instance, arresting someone, as Punch points out, can be seen as a failure to negotiate the outcome in terms of 'service' work. The police manual instructs the police to make all efforts at persuasion. A value is placed on the skill of 'smoothing things over' and achieving some arrangement 'to take care of the problem'.

It is Punch's contention that the police occupational ideology of hostile stereotypes of other agencies brings them into conflict with such agencies and, in particular, with social workers. However, the present study does not support Punch's picture of 'continuing conflict, competition and confusion'.[27] Rather, the police have been found to be ready users of the psychiatric option, particularly if hospitalisation can also be interpreted as confinement. Psychiatric hospitalisation is clearly a most useful resource for the police in their task of tidying-up social troubles. In this respect, the police operate in the same way as social workers, viewing hospital admission as an effective solution which disposes of a problem in a 'caring response'.

Conflict arises, however, when the psychiatric services seek to maintain ideological purity and resist hospitalisation. The strategies invoked by the hospital gatekeepers - the psychiatrists- will be discussed after the role of the other chief agent of social control - the social workers - is examined.

Notes

1. Scheff, T. (1964) 'The Societal Reation to Deviance' Ascriptive Elements in the Psychiatric Screening of Patients in a Mid-Western State', *Social Problems*, 11, pp. 401-13.
2. Department of Health and Social Services, Hospital Statistics (1979) report a figure of 12 per cent compulsory admissions in England.
3. Miller, K., Simons, R. and Fein, S. (1974) 'Compulsory Mental Hospitalisation in England and Wales', *Journal of Health and Social Behaviour*, 15, pp. 151-56. The authors report a figure of 19 per cent formal admissions over the period 1965-70.
4. Ibid. Miller et al found a range of 10 per cent variation between regions, groups and over time.
5. Miles, H., Loudon, J. and Rawnsley, K. (1960) 'Attitudes and Practices of Mental Welfare Officers' *Public Health*, 76, pp. 32-47.
6. Coie, J., Costanza, R. and Cox, G. (1975) 'Behavioural Determinants of Mental Illness Concerns, *Journal of Consulting and Clinical Psychology*, 43, pp. 626-36. The authors studied the attitudes of five 'gatekeeping' groups towards mental illness and found the policy particularly sensitive and knowledgeable about labelling in these borderline areas.
7. Ibid.
8. Hollingshead, A. and Redlich, F. (1958) *Social Class and Mental Illness*, New York. The authors found that in the lowest socioeconomic class, more than half of psychotic patients were referred by the police. Hsu, U.F. 'Police Co-Operation in Connection with Mental Cases in Peiping', in *Neuropsychiatry in China*, eds. Lyman, R., Maeker, V. and Liang, P. (1939) p. 203 - Police commital was primarily concerned with labourers, soldiers and the police themselves.
9. Scheff, T. (1975) *Labelling Madness*, New Jersey.

Gove, W. (1980) *The Labelling of Deviance*, London.

10. Rushing, W. (1971) 'Individual Resources, Societal Reaction and Hospital Commitment', *American Journal of Sociology*, 77, pp. 511-26. Gove, W. and Howell, P. (1974) 'Individual Resources and Mental Hospitalisation'. A Comparison and Evaluation of the Societal Reaction and Psychiatric Perspectives', 39, pp. 86-100. Myers, J. and Roberts, B. (1959) *Famly and Class Dynamics in Mental Illness*, New York. Hollingshead, A. and Redlich, F. (1958) op. cit.
11. Bean, P. (1980) *Compulsory Admission to Mental Hospitals*, Chichester.
12. Liberman, R. (1969) 'Police as a Community Mental Health Resource', *Community Mental Health Journal*, 5, p. 11120.
13. Horowitz, A. (1977) 'Social Networks to Pathways to Psychiatric Treatment', *Social Forces*, 56, pp. 86-105. Those living alone will only come to attention in public places when their disordered behaviour draws the attention of the authorities. It is suggested by Horowitz that those with closed networks, suffer a more prolonged deterioration of behaviour that requires police involvement to achieve hospital admission.
14. Benson, D. and Hughes, J. (1983) *The Perspective of Ethnomethodology*, Essex.
15. The Police Manual only lays down guidelines as to their responsibility to escort a patient to hospital. It says nothing as to how to handle disturbed behaviour in public places.
16. Punch, M. (1979) 'The Secret Social Service' in Holdaway, A. *The British Police*, London. Punch foundt hat over half the routine calls to the police involved demands for help and some form of support for personal and interpersonal problems.
17. Bittner, E. 'Police Discrimination in the Emergency Apprenhension of Mentally Ill Persons'. In Douglas, J. eds *Introduction to Deviance*. The author found that the police engaged in five forms of denial: that they had insufficient evidence; that it would only burden the hospital to the limit of its capacity; that dealing with the mentally ill is not a proper task for them; that it is a tedious and uncertain procedure that did not necessarily lead to a tidy solution; and a general reluctance to get people locked up with the rest of the 'crazies'. There was local evidence of this last form of denial from a policeman who told me he 'shrank from putting people in'.
18. Coie, J. et al (1975) op cit., found a difference between urban and rural police; the former being more tolerant and basing their judgement about personal inappropriateness upon their personal knowledge of the person.
19. A policeman described the process as one of saying 'leave it with us' and then going away and forgetting about it after listening to 'a load of old rubbish'.
20. Mendel, W. 'Determinants of the Decision for Psychiatric Hospitalisation', *Archives General Psychiatry*, 20, pp. 321-8.
21. Hsu, F. (1939) op. cit.
22. Bittner, E., op. cit. 'Keeping the Peace' is described as 'an occupational routine with particular procedures, skills, standards, and information which meets public expectations'.
23. Punch, M. op. cit.
24. Bittner, E. op. cit.

25. Clausen, J.A. and Yarrow, M.R. (1955) 'Paths to the Mental Hospital', *Journal of Social Issues*, 11, pp. 25-32: A study of the ways in which the husbands of 33 wives became psychiatric patients.
26. Punch, M. op. cit.
27. Ibid.

9 The social worker

Social workers act as labellers in the social process of psychiatric hospitalisation. They have legal authority to apply for compulsory admission in place of nearest relative. As a social worker in a psychiatric hospital I worked as part of this system and was involved in making decisions about the admission, care, discharge and support of patients. In this chapter I intend to describe this activity from the perspective of a participant. I will be reporting on my own decision-making and on the values, motives and ideology that informed such decisions.

I became a social worker in a psychiatric hospital partly out of curiosity about a group of people who had been 'glamourised' as deviants in the counter culture of the seventies and described as underdogs. These ideas derived primarily from the work of R. D. Laing[1] who had constructed an alternative perspective by listening to patients' accounts of their mental illness developing from relationships in their families. Such a perspective was particularly attractive to social work as it offered an alternative to the medical model. It also emphasised the need for intervention in an area in which social workers operated, and utilised one of the methods of social work, listening to people talk. However, Laing's ideas had not made the journey from the university library to the county psychiatric hospital where his name was never mentioned and the 'anti-psychiatry' school of thought was viewed with hostility.

It quickly became apparent to me in my work in the hospital that these people who were psychiatric patients did not seem very different from those people I had known as clients as a community social worker. Those clients had never been anywhere near a psychiatric hospital and it had never entered my head to consider hospital admission as a solution to their enormous problems. This began my interest in the question of how people became hospital patients.

Social Work as a Profession

The establishment of social workers in psychiatric hospitals developed out of the American sponsorship of Child Guidance Clinics with psychiatric social workers employed as psychotherapists and trained in a psychodynamic model. Such staff were few and most people entered the posts of hospital almoner and Mental Welfare Officers with no formal training.[2] MWOs operated in the community with a statutory responsibility to bring persons to hospital, and they developed practical and pragmatic approaches to their work.[3] The way in which they operated was largely influenced by administrative factors and institutional contingencies. The Seebohm Report brought about the amalgamation in the early 1970s, of these posts under the umbrella of social services departments. A system of uniform generic training was introduced which, it was hoped, would promote a shared set of values and a professional identity.

Social work has been described as a 'semi-profession' in that it lacks the autonomy and status of the fully-fledged professions.[4] It has particular characteristics because social workers are professional employees of the government and operate in bureaucratic structures. State mediation in the form of Social Services Departments has brought bureaucracy and a likely conflict between organisational rules and procedures, and the values of the profession. Social work values are grounded in the techniques of psychotherapy and as such they offer little of practical value to the social worker operating in the middle ground between the individual and society. Their value system has been described as empty and has been ridiculed.[5] The decision-making involved in the practical day-to-day activity of social work derives from common-sense theorising as much as from the idea of social work as psychotherapy.[6]

The particular features of social work in a psychiatric hospital revolve around the need to mediate between the patient and/or his family on the one side and the hospital on the other. For the hospital social worker, the hospital is in many ways the society against which the needs of the individual are mediated. The experience of social workers in working with families is recognised by the psychiatrist who employs the social worker to investigate the patient's family background.

A feature of hospital social work is social control. The social worker is vested with the authority to sign someone into hospital in the absence, or with the approval of the nearest relative.[8] It has been found that social workers have a higher tolerance of deviant behaviour than other gatekeeper groups which could be attributed to their familiarity with deviance and disorder.[9] On the other hand, there may be a mutual antipathy between referring doctor and social worker[10]. Legislation requires that it be ascertained that all alternatives to hospital should be investigated and it has been suggested (by a psychiatrist) that social workers are in the best position to know the range of resources.[11]

Such tasks are in the nature of 'dirty work' in that not being able to do something for clients in the therapeutic sense, the social worker is required to do something <u>to</u> them in a coercive sense.[12] The social worker may take care to distance himself from such activity in order to retain his professional integrity. But the whole of social work activity has been characterised in similar vein as society's dustbin men clearing up the detritus of humanity.[13]

Because of the contradiction between professional ideology and daily work social workers engage in considerable rationalisation and accommodation. An example of this is the way frustrations with work are sometimes internalised into personal inadequacies or shortcomings.

Psychiatrists' Expectations of Social Workers

Psychiatrists have been strongly critical of the reorganisation of social work which has removed the 'hand-maiden' of the psychiatric social worker with allegiance to and training in the psychiatric model. In a survey of opinion, some 77 per cent of psychiatrists felt that the quality of social work service had deteriorated as a result of Seebohm reorganisation and they can still be heard to bemoan the passing of the specialist worker.[14] Their dissatisfaction centres on the removal of the social worker from their sphere of influence and his allegiance to alternative perspectives on mental illness.[15]

Social workers fill a subsidiary role to the psychiatrist and in this position have passed on to them the less pleasant and more stigmatising work that the psychiatrist does not wish to perform.[16] Psychiatrists justify the devolving of such (from their point of view) demeaning responsibilities in terms of the particular skills of social workers. This offers a ready made rationalisation to social work for the undertaking of such tasks. There are two particular areas of responsibility : the first is work with patients who have been described as 'not mentally ill' and fit into the 'undeserving ' category[17]; the second is the management of conflict when a doctor recommends the admission of someone to hospital against their will.[18]

One of the chief functions that the psychiatrist requires of the social worker is the collection of information from the family and others about the patient's background and previous activities from which information a biography may be constructed. The skill of the social worker is described as the ability 'to recognise the likelihood of the presence of mental illness even where the symptoms appear in the form of social problems, and where the client has not been in touch with the medical services'.[19] In this task of re-interpretation, the social worker takes the information supplied from relatives, and reinterprets aspects into descriptions of behaviour that the psychiatrist may identify as symptomatology.

Re-interpreting Activity

The social worker brings to the task of re-interpretation his 'technical' language with which he translates the account of everyday events collected from relatives into a 'scientised' body of knowledge. One of the reasons why professionals engage in such activity is the opportunity for 'mystification' by which the professional is able to display his technical abilities. This task has particular problems for social workers for two reasons: firstly, the material which social workers rework is peculiarly ordinary and everyday; secondly, social work has itself some commitment to 'demystify' professional activity.

The theoretical base of social work is made up of three components. Firstly the discipline developed out of the activities of a group of psychotherapeutic practitioners who sought a distinct professional identity. Their theoretical background was psychoanalysis and they analysed their work in terms of psychotherapeutic and analytical concepts. Secondly, alongside the acquisition of responsibilities for the delivery of welfare services, social workers became concerned with how society works and adopted sociological concepts to describe the phenomena with which they were confronted in their daily work. Thirdly, social workers were empowered by the state with responsibilities to protect the welfare of the vulnerable and adopted the phrases from the Acts to describe their activity.[19]

Re-interpreting activity deals with conflict situations and translates such conflict into a form of deviance, in this case mental illness. When the social worker makes this translation he will try to avoid making a moral judgement. This is because the values of social work brought from psychotherapy allow for description but not judgement.[20] Family conflict is neutralised into analytical terms like projection and displacement. Interpersonal relationships are described in terms of the feelings involved, for instance and most commonly, by overprotection and over-dependence. The concept of stress has been adopted to link extraneous influences to the individual. Social-psychological concepts of group activity in the family can be used to focus on relationships such as 'scapegoating'.

The second method of description is sociological and may well contain political judgement. Conflict, in this case, is conceptualised in terms of social deprivation, and more extremely as class domination. Socio-cultural explanations, may also be adopted. Other sociological concepts frequently used are the concept of role, and the concept of stigma to describe lack of family tolerance.

The most common term in use is the concept of coping or managing. Social workers make decisions about the ability of clients to cope on their own, to manage their home, to cope with their children, to care for an elderly relative, and so on. If the client is not able to cope then their dependents are described as 'at risk', or in the phrase of the Children's Act 'in need of care and attention'. Being 'at risk' or 'in need of care' are terms that are frequently used by social workers to justify their intervention in situations against their clients' wishes. These terms are at the opposite end of the spectrum from the values of psychotherapy and are functionally important as justifications of acts of social control.

Interviews with families of patients often have a dual purpose for the hospital social worker. The psychiatrist may have requested background information, a 'social history' of the patient. At the same time, the social worker will be concerned to establish a casework relationship independently of the psychiatrist. There are problems with doing both simultaneously; the collection of information often cuts across the expression of feelings. In some ways interviewing relatives for 'social histories' can be essentially similar to interviewing patients for symptomatology. The social worker is aware of the sort of information of interest to the psychiatrist, and asks his questions accordingly. An important feature of psychiatric interviews is the significance of 'key terms'. In an amorphous mass of information the mention of particular items act as 'releaser cues'. These concentrate the enquiry on a particular area of behaviour and release the use of a predictable and specific set of questions.[21] For instance, a comment from a relative about a patient 'feeling very low' releases a series of questions about sleep, weight, appetite, guilt, and self-harm. The social worker may well be more interested in feelings of loss and bereavement but is sensitive to the collection of such information that the psychiatrist can re-interpret into evidence of symptoms of mental illness.

Two other important areas of inquiry are, firstly, the relative's description of the patient's previous personality what is termed the 'pre-morbid' personality. Out of such phrases as 'she was always a worrier' are constructed for the psychiatrist an image of the former person which the psychiatrist conceptualises as a 'base line' on which to judge recovery. Secondly, information about history of mental illness in the patient's family is of great interest to the psychiatrist who may well use it as a defining characteristic in the diagnosing of mental illness.

The psychiatrist is essentially concerned to transform patient's behaviour from conflict to illness. This involves locating the source of trouble within the individual rather than in his general situation. Psychiatrists are reluctant to let the social world intrude but prefer to view the patients' condition as akin to a morbid anatomy. If there is too much information, the psychiatrist finds it difficult to diagnose. From his point of view, 'social histories' are a means to provide evidence of symptoms and to enable diagnosis.

Management of Conflict

Bean reports that psychiatrists regard compulsory admission as 'at worst, a necessary evil, and, at best, an area of professional practice which produces moral doubts.'[22] There is some evidence that psychiatrists may seek to deny this 'dirty work' and to pass on responsibility for its management to social workers.[23] Social workers are expected to protect the rights and liberty of the patient from the position of an 'emergent profession, that has yet to establish its credibility in this field'.[25] As an emergent profession, social work has taken on such impossible tasks, seeing in them an opportunity to expand its area of expertise.[25] The inherent contradictions are denied in the attempt to reconcile duties of social control with individual self-determination. The way in which social workers have dealt with such paradoxes is best illustrated by examples.

Local Social Service Departments are primarily concerned with ensuring that young children are adequately cared for. Their involvement in mental hospital admission is often a consequence of their concern for adequate care of the children of the patient.[26]

> 'R' had looked after her children for many years and her care of them was monitored by a social worker. She relied on her husband who deserted her for several months at a time. He was foreign and R. had identified with his culture and community and rejected her own family. When her husband failed to return, 'R' left the housework, and did not restrain the children's behaviour. As a

> result, her neighbours complained about their lack of supervision and about her immodest dress. Neighbours also described 'R' as being 'in a world of her own'. When 'R' refused her child treatment after an accident, steps were taken to remove her children into the care of social services.

'R's capabilities to care on her own for her children were clearly in question. A psychiatrist was asked to visit her at home and advised admission. In hospital, her identification with a foreign culture and, her claim to speak that language when being heard listening to different foreign station, provided items of behaviour to be interpreted as a delusional system. This positive symptomatology was combined with the negative symptomatology of self neglect and apathy into a diagnosis of severe mental illness. Her family provided details of her biography ready for reworking; her marginality was both evidence of her social drift and identified as the reason why she had avoided admission for treatment of her mental illness.

This case illustrates the nature of the social work concern. 'R's behaviour is only assessed when the future care of her children has to be decided. Her social worker sees little difference in her throughout this period, before and after treatment. Here is a second example of the social worker in action.

> As hospital social worker, I had been involved with 'J' and his discharge from a long-stay ward to hostel accommodation. However, after a few weeks in the hostel, 'J' refused to pay the hostel rent and was aggressive to the hostel supervisor. He was discharged from the hostel but refused to see a doctor and returned home to live with his parents. At the sheltered workshop where he worked, he gave himself a different name and claimed to be married. His family tolerated him at home but complained about his 'taking over'. He refused to pay his mother for his keep and got drunk in the city where he went to find his 'wife'. 'J' stopped his tablets, stayed in bed till afternoon and watched the T.V. news all the time laughing unexpectedly.

Each of these behaviours can be interpreted as symptoms of a relapse of his mental illness. The extent to which I engaged in such reinterpretation (and encouraged the family to do likewise) is influenced by my attitudes and determined by my 'rules of thumb'. Straddling the hospital and family the social worker's own judgement of what is acceptable behaviour is crucial.He stands in a position of authority as a 'professional' to provide an 'expert' opinion, and thereby influence the attitudes of J.'s family towards him. There is an expectation of the social worker to provide a solution and one such solution the family is likely to expect is hospital admission. In order to keep such an option open, the social worker is unlikely to jepordise his working relationship with the hospital doctors by confrontation. For pragmatic reasons he is likely not to reveal any belief in the labelling perspective or a lack of faith in the medical model. The resolution of crises is a daily task for the social worker, which depends on good relations with those occupations that control access to scarce resources.[27]

Hospital admission means that the responsibility for 'J' will be passed on to the hospital. This is an attractive solution compared with finding 'J' a place in another hostel, a more 'arduous' task for the social worker. Such a 'disposal' would require the social worker to keep responsibility and ensure 'J's welfare. Hospital admission can also be justified in terms of 'time-out' from breaking human relationships. For 'J' the price will be tablets and injections.

Such reasoning assumed that 'J' would agree to come into hospital which in fact, he did not. He stayed at home and his mother 'juggled' the situation by acceding to his demands in order to keep the peace. Another out-patient appointment was arranged in the hope of hospital readmission. My thinking had three strands: that being a social recluse is socially unhealthy and should be discouraged; that 'J's quality of life would improve in hospital; and most importantly, that his mother could not cope with him and needed protection from 'J's demands.

'J' was physically aggressive to his mother one night and the police were called, but left when his mother did not press charges. The G.P. would not visit because the family had moved out of his area. The hospital would not admit 'J' without a G.P.'s recommendation. It was a weekend night and his mother waited till Monday to see me. She showed her injuries; the younger children were afraid to stay in the house. It was up to the social worker to get 'J' into hospital because he was a risk to the family. His former G.P. was contacted, who arranged a home visit. 'J's symptoms were earmarked : his sudden attack was unpredictable and aggressive; his laughing at the television was evidence of incongruity; his staying in the house was social withdrawal; his belief that he had a wife and that his mother was someone else were delusions. The G.P. called to the house and arranged a compulsory admission.

This case shows the importance of the social worker in resolving a conflict situation by describing behaviour in a particular way and by his access to the 'gatekeepers'. He is able to influence the course of events by deciding at what stage to intervene and in what way. In practical terms, these issues boil down to realities such as pressure from family and the level of perceived risk to others from the patient's behaviour.

The 'Undeserving'

This category of patient is usually in hospital for a minimum period during which attempts are made to 'demedicalise' his behaviour. Doctors often take an authoritative approach and insist to the patient that he is not ill. However, the ramifications and consequences of such a person's behaviour may well become the concern of the social worker. This may occur on the social worker's own initiative and be bound up with his responsibilities towards protecting other vulnerable groups from disruptive behaviour. Duties towards the family of the patient will fall into this category. Hospital admission can be viewed as a quick and effective resolution of a crisis, but it is often only a short-term solution.

The social worker performs an important function in picking up the social consequences of hospital admission. Doctors are preoccupied with not 'blocking beds'; the social worker has to mobilise alternatives to avoid prolonged hospitalisation, and to show that a caring response has been made so that discharge may follow. In this way the social worker is used by the psychiatrist to pick up on work that he regards as inappropriate. In return the social worker may reasonably expect the psychiatrist to help him and his colleagues out of difficulties and offer a hospital bed when requested. By such methods crises are defused and people are handled.

Of particular interest is the transfer of a patient from the status of a 'deserving' case with a 'genuine' mental illness to the status of an 'undeserving' patient who is required to take responsibility for his actions. Such transformations are a recent feature of hospital life but are becoming more frequent as doctors seek to refine their classifications. To achieve such redefinitions the psychiatrist leans heavily upon the social worker who is sometimes required to explain to the patient's family the new diagnosis and to spell out the consequences.The dynamics involved are best illustrated by example.

> 'B' has been a problem for his parents since he became a teenager; they have brought him through the spectrum of 'helping agencies' but his behaviour remains beyond their control. This behaviour has been redefined with each new assessment: from behaviour disorder in the child psychiatry clinic, to problem child in the children's home, to delinquent in the training school. 'B' has been admitted to psychiatric hospital and redefined as mentally ill. His biography has been reworked to provide evidence of symptomatology. For example, his allegory of himself as a tiger in the jungle, previously viewed as fantasy, was reinterpreted as delusion.

The medicalisation of 'B's behaviour made his family feel responsible and made conflict more acceptable as the symptoms of a mental illness. Being sick, B. is no longer responsible for the disruptions that he caused. However, as 'B's behaviour is not affected by medication, there is increasing pressure to change his diagnosis. The process of removal of the previously ascribed label of illness means the loss of the privileges of the sick role. The social consequences to patient and family are far-reaching. The social worker is in the middle of the re-negotiation that must take place. B. is told that he is now responsible for his actions and his family are required to support this notion.

The extent to which exit from the sick role is achieved will be determined by factors in the wider situation. For the psychiatrist his change of opinion needs to be passed on to his medical colleagues who act as gatekeepers. The doctor sees discharge as the cut-off point for the hospital but those outside involved with B. are likely to cling to the medical model and seek further hospital admission as a resolution to the problem.

It falls to the social worker to mobilise alternatives which may well not exist. Although the police cling to the psychiatric label they are informed otherwise by the social worker. B. was inducted into the criminal justice system , first on probation, then in detention centre and finally in prison. Such is the way morality is re-established; Thomas Szasz would approve. But even in jail there is still the possibility that B. will be reassessed by the attached psychiatrist and achieve re-entry to the psychiatric patient role.

It can be seen that entry and exit into and out of the psychiatric patient role is not a straightforward affair but one that involves frequent overlap between 'gatekeeper' groups. The degree to which the mental illness label represents a master status for the individual[28] is determined by the interplay between the involved professional groups. Whether the patient's family accepts such reworking seems to be of lesser importance.

In such activity it falls to the social worker to play a crucial role. Whilst the delabelling of a young person and his release from hospital would, prima facie, seem an act to be welcomed, the lack of alternatives to hospital make the reality rather grim.

Rules of Thumb for Social Workers

The way in which social workers are involved in the labelling of mental illness is influenced by two main issues. These are the nature of psychiatric emergencies as crises and the concern of the social worker for the wider situation.

The management of crisis requires certain 'people handling skills'.[29] Social workers' perceptions of mental illness may well conform to the public stereotype and they are just as likely to be fearful of violence. People who become social workers do not usually have the training, physique or attitude to deal with violent people. They must rely on their ability to 'cool things down', to be 'a still centre' in dangerous or potentially dangerous situations.[30] Common sense techniques are used such as speaking in a slow and calm voice, and sitting down to appear less threatening. Conversation is 'neutral' and concerned with everyday events. Social workers differ perceptibly from other labelling groups, such as doctors and the police, in that they do not possess the same degree of vested authority. In his ordinary work with people the strategy of the social worker is one of alignment, a suggestion to the client - 'I am on your side'. This position may carry the implication that the social worker cares more than the other professionals and has more integrity. Such positioning originates in the philanthropic activities of early social work which surfaced in a sympathy for the underdog. When the social worker is required to do something to his client against his wishes rather than for him, then he is in conflict with his social work ideology. He may engage in role distance to resolve this dilemna.[31]

Mental illness has been seen as both a residual category and a stigmatised status. As such, it is only used as a last resort when other alternatives are exhausted. People only resort to such a drastic solution when they are desperate. Desperate situations present as crises demanding resolution, usually at night and weekends. The easiest resolution, the most immediate and most effective, is removal of the culprit, the person who is being blamed as the trouble-maker. There are relatively few options open for removal and any social worker is motivated by a need to keep such options open. Perhaps the most convenient is psychiatric hospitalisation which is viewed as a solution since the offender, the cause of the trouble, has been removed. The alternative of removal by the police involves the criminalisation of behaviour, a solution which fits badly with the values of social work.[32] In contrast, the sick role is a partly legitimised status with less attendant stigma. Being mentally ill is a stigmatised status but short term admission may not carrry the same connotations. By such rationalisations, decisions are justified.

The chief contrast between the social worker and the psychiatrist is in the nature of their concerns: the social worker is concerned with what social work ideology defines as "the total situation" whilst the psychiatrist is primarily concerned with that person identified as patient. Because his concern is the functioning of the family as a whole, the social worker is more amenable to family pressure.[33] It is the social worker who will be visiting the family home once the patient leaves hospital, and he will seek to ensure that the family will tolerate the patient's return home. Because of these differences in concerns the social worker's perspective may seem somewhat misplaced to the psychiatrist. Such misunderstandings are sometimes characteristic of the multi-disciplinary team 'in action' in the psychiatric hospital.

Notes

1. Laing, R. and Esterson, A. (1964) *'Sanity Madness and the Family'*, Harmondsworth. The authors describe the dynamics of eleven families from which a child had been diagnosed schizophrenic.
   Laing, R. (1960) *'The Divided Self'*, London.
2. Miles, H., Loudon, J. and Rawnsley, K. (1960) 'Attitudes and Practice of Mental Welfare Officers', *Public Health*, 76, pp. 32-47. The authors quote a figure of 60 per cent of M.W.O.'s having no qualifications whatsoever.
3. Lawson, A. (1966) *Mental Illness in London.* Maudsley Monograph No. 15, London. A study of the Mental Welfare Department in London and their decision-making found that 'the social policies, aministrative apparatus and other attendant nosocomical factors had the greatest influence on the course of events.
4. Etzioni, A. (1969) *The Semi-Professions and Their Organisation*, London.
5. Pearson, G. (1975) 'Making Social Workers' in *Radical Social Work* edidted by Bailey, R. and Brake, M., London. Pearson quotes W.G. Auden: 'Writers can be guilty of every kind of conceit but one, the conceit of the social worker - we are all here on earth to help others: what on earth the others are here for I don't know'.
6. Mayer, J. and Timms, N. (1970) *The Client Speaks*, A study of clients' reports of social worker contact in which a high level of misunderstanding was found due to the social worker using psychodynamic, non-directive methods when the working-class client expected material help and a directive approach.
7. Oram, E. (1977) 'The Making of a Mental Welfare Officer' *Community Care*, March 23, 1977. To quote '...a generalised family casework skill which is able to recognise those family and environmental tensions which lead to the disruption of normal living and which result in a member of the group exhibiting disturbed behaviour which labels him as the 'patient'.
8. Mental Health Act (N.I.) 1961, Section 13.

9. Coie, J., Costanza, P. and Cox, G. (1975) 'Behavioural Determinants of Mental Illness Concerns: A Comparison of 'Gatekeeper' Professions, *Journal of Consulting and Clinical Psychology*, 43, pp. 626-36.
   Bean, P. (1980) *Compulsory Admissions to Mental Hospital*, London, p. 157.
10. Ibid. The author found relationships of professional rivalry bordering on hostility between social workers and psychiatrists.
11. Oram, E. (1977) op. cit.
12. Emerson, R. and Pollner, M. (1976) 'Dirty Work Designations: Their Features in a Psychiatric Setting'. *Social Problems*, pp. 243-54.
13. Cohen, S. (1975) 'Manifestoes in Action' in *Radical Social Work* edited by Bailey, R. and Brake, M, London.
14. Little, J. and Burkitt, E. 'Psychiatry and the Social Worker', *S K and F Publications*. This survey of psychiatrists' opinions reports that 77 per cent of psychiatrists thought that the social work service had deteriorated post-Seebohm, although pre-Seebohm nearly half the sample described social work service as 'average', implying a degree of reservation if not dissatisfaction.
15. Ibid. p. 29. 'No man can serve two masters. Social Workers have forsaken us and cling to their departments'.
16. Etzioni, A. (1969) op. cit. quoting Everett Hughes:' One way in which professionals dispense of unpleasant tasks is to define them as sub-professional and assign them to less favoured groups. The professional group carrying them then attempts to redefine them and to invest them with professional dignity and importance'.
17. Oram, E. (1977) op. cit. p. 24. 'They (social workers) do much to alleviate the sense of outrage which such victims feel about the diagnosis made about them. Psychiatrists are most appreciative of social workers who give relief to these troubled persons with disturbed emotional reactions, but who show no symptoms of psychiatric illness'.
18. Ibid. p. 24. 'A social worker should be able to create a relationship with the patient and relatives, and establish the problem as a medical or a social matter, rather than a behaviour problem, and where necessary introduce the doctors to a more controlled environment where they may freely express their considered professional opinions'.
19. Children's and Young Person's Act (N.I.) 1968
   Health and Personal Social Services Order (N.I.) 1972.
20. Biestek, F. (1961) *The Casework Relationship*, London. The author identifies seven core principles of social work: individualisation, purposeful expression of feelings; controlled emotional involement; acceptance; non-judgemental attitude; client self-determination; and confidentiality.
21. Bean, P. (1980) op. cit. Bean lists the key terms in two levels of importance: at the upper level are terms and phrases such as 'hearing voices', 'thinking of suicide', 'loss of weight', 'sleeplessness', etc. At a lower level were 'unhappy', 'miserable', 'frightened', or 'upset'.
22. Ibid, p. 129.

23. Oram, E. (1977) op. cit. 'Where compulsion becomes necessary the aim should be to effect admission with no more distress than any other form of illness'.
24. Ibid, p. 23.
25. Bean, P. (1980) op. cit: The author found that social workers in England, in nearly all cases, acted as surrogate relative in formalising patients to hospital when the Act requires them to only do so when the relative is unavailable or unwilling to sign, but raises no objection to the social worker doing so.
26. In the present study, those admissions where social servicse personnel were the referral agent divided as follows: 50 per cent of cases involved a social worker with child-care concerns mobilising psychiatric care for the mother; other referrals were made up of residential staff who could not manage an elderly resident. There were also two cases of hostel staff initiating referral of young ex-patients.
27. Good working relations with the police are useful to the social worker who may require their assistance to remove children at risk in the middle of the night. Police in return expect social worker's co-operation in admission to psychiatric hospital.
28. Scheff, T. (1975) *Labelling Madness*, New Jersey. Scheff postulates that being labelled mentally ill creates a master status for the individual that then determines, in a large measure, the nature of interaction to which the individual is subject.
29. Butler, A. and Pritchard, C. (1983) *Social Work and Mental Illness*, London.
30. Prins, H. (1980) *Offenders, Deviants or Patients*, London. The author advises on how social workers should manage violent situations.
31. Goffman, E. (1972) *Encounters: Two Studies in the Sociology of Interaction*, London.
32. The police frequently justify their referrals to social services in terms of 'their hands are tied' because people cannot be kept in a cell overnight without being charged.
33. Miles, H. et al. (1960) report that 'family circumstances played an important part with all officers in assisting them to decide what course to take'.

10 The psychiatrist

Although some pattern has emerged amongst the social variables identified in the patient population it has been seen that the way in which people arrive in hospital is almost fortuitous. The behaviours that people bring to hospital are often so diverse as to resist distillation but it is the task of the psychiatrist to try to do so. The number of patients and the pressure of time make this a difficult proposition.

People arrive in hospital on the basis of lay definitions of behaviour; family, police, social workers and neighbours are variously involved in this process. In the process of becoming patients, people pass through a 'mortification of self'[1] before filling their new, stigmatised status. As patients, they are the subject of investigation and labelling by the hospital staff led by the psychiatrist. The fact of being in hospital almost certainly results in a label of mental illness: in only one instance, during the research period, was the description 'not psychiatrically ill' applied.[2] The psychiatrist diagnoses what the public bring to hospital and he is able to influence public opinion about what constitutes mental illness by his defining activity.[3] This is a symbiotic relationship which is fluid, for as attitudes liberalise, behaviour previously judged unacceptable becomes tolerated.[4] Social values and ideological considerations in society are important variables influencing the nature of psychiatrists' activity.

The judgements of psychiatrists are the outcome of the interaction between their own beliefs and values and the beliefs and expectations of the wider society. The process of decision-making contains elements of conflict and contradiction between current psychiatric theory, the meaning of mental illness for the psychiatrist, the social meaning of mental illness, the meaning of mental illness for the patient, and the nature of psychiatric facilities as a scarce resource. Decisions are made on the basis of a shared socially accredited body of knowledge in so far as there is agreement on what it contains. The use of these concepts is governed by a set of rules .

Professional Ideology

In Northern Ireland, psychiatry remains closely attached to the field of medicine; it is a specialism contained under the medical umbrella. Psychiatrists view themselves as doctors first and foremost. The professional characteristics of psychiatry are therefore those of medicine in general. The characteristics of the medical profession have been described as collegiate, autonomous, and self-governing. A strong peer solidarity is promoted through journals, conferences, a common, technical language, and an occupational ideology that emphasises practice. As medical students, all doctors share a common student culture, a period of socialisation and training that continues for six years[5]. Medical students are drawn from a small stratum of society; in Northern Ireland sons and daughters frequently follow fathers into medicine. Father and sons, and husband and wife practices are not uncommon. Drawn from an elite in a traditional society, kinship and friendship bonds bind together doctors into a closed and privileged group.

The medical profession has successfully argued for its own control of its activity through the British Medical Association. In medicine a homogenous occupational group enjoys a large demand from a heterogeneous consumer group, leaving the latter dependent and exploitable. The authority of the doctor is high in the one to one relationships that pertain.[6] The medical profession argues that the potential for abuse is held in check by the ideal of service, promulgated by the profession. But as technology advances and medical expertise becomes more specialised, the patient is left more mystified. Parsons argued that informal mechanisms prevent abuse but it may well be that the increase in medical activity and the expansion in the authority of the doctor have swamped such restraints.[7]

After six years in medical school it is inevitable that the allegiance of the prospective psychiatrist is to the medical model of mental illness. This model initiates in imitation of general medicine in which conditions are seen as separate and discrete entities and constellations of symptoms indicate diagnosis.[8] One of the basic divisions is between the affective psychoses which are cyclical and which may well get better eventually without treatment, and the schizophrenias which are sporadic and leave a residual element.[9] However, one of the most difficult things for the psychiatrist is to fit the reality he encounters into a strict scientific classificatory system. This is one of the central themes of psychiatrists' decision-making.

There is not the same allegiance to the medical model in America where 80 per cent of psychiatrists described their orientation as psychotherapeutic.[10] American psychiatry accommodates widely differing perspectives on a continuum from directive-organic to analytic-psychological. It seems reasonable to anticipate that values and social background should be linked to orientation. Psychotherapy entrants have been found to be similar - Jewish-European and liberal.[11] On the other hand, dislike of emotionally disturbed patients has been linked to dogmatic and authoritarian personality traits.[12, 13]

Ulster psychiatrists share the middle class background of their compatriots in general medicine. In England, emergency psychiatry has been described as a 'high class occupation aimed at low class personnel'.[14] The psychiatrist makes judgements about normal and abnormal behaviour on the basis of his own cultural background. This is likely to be very different from the cultural background of his patient. Judgements may be made on the basis of cultural values that are alien to the context in which the behaviour being judged occurs. Alternatively, psychiatrists may guess about how the social class of their patients behaves. Judgements of conduct and behaviour contain a subjective element with the result that psychiatrists may differ amongst themselves in their diagnoses[15].

Psychiatry is an eclectic discipline which has accommodated social and psychological explanations as subsidiary explanations. An example of this intellectual imperialism is the incorporation of Laing and Esterson's highlighting of family dysfunction as a factor in schizophrenia[16] into the measurement of high expressed emotion as developed by Vaughn and Leff.[17] Medical students are alerted to measure the amount of critical and over-emotionally involved acts directed against a person with schizophrenia by his family. Within the psychiatric hospital 'pardigm clashes' do not openly occur.[18] In the wider society the position and ideas of psychiatry are only cautiously accepted, but within the psychiatric hospital the medical perspective is firmly entrenched.

Non-medical staff (psychologists and social workers) seldom have the same allegiance to the medical model and may even hold opposing beliefs. However, direct ideological confrontation is unusual, and each discipline continues to do 'its own thing'. There is a compartmentalism of ideas similar to that which exists among patients. The patient engages in 'double entry book-keeping' by which he does not believe he is ill but will continue to take tablets ; the psychiatrist believes in mental disorder as illness but will emphasise social causation; and the social worker seeks to avoid labelling but attends wards rounds.

There are three aspects to the professional ideology of psychiatrists. In the first place, their allegiance is to medicine and they share its commitment to service. In the second place, they are strongly committed to the act of diagnosing and to the classificatory system of mental illness although the fitting of concrete reality into a strict scientific model causes them enormous difficulties. In the third place, like any other occupational group they are commited to the preservation and strengthening of their profession.

Society's Expectations of Psychiatrists

Today psychiatric hospital were bequeathed by the Victorians. Foucault suggests that one of their motives was a need to classify the lower classes into employability.[20] Originally called asylums, they were controlled by Superintendents until medicine took over during the nineteenth century. They remained places of containment until medical discoveries such as E.C.T. in the 1930s and tranquilliser drugs in the 1950s. With the development of psychopharmocological methods, there were hopes that the psychiatric hospitals would be emptied of patients.

There are two reasons why developments have not, as anticipated, cleared the mental hospitals. Firstly, as the profession has sought to strengthen and expand it has made over-ambitious claims for new developments. Psychiatry has tended to over-praise its achievements and collude with a public who see medicine as the panacea to all troubles. Secondly, psychiatry has in the past tended to medicalise new areas of human activity. Ivan Illich has spoken out vehemently against this medicalisation of life and believes medicine itself to be the fastest growing cause of disease.[21] For example, the classificatory system of mental illnesses has developed into a glossary that included rating keys for behaviours such as lesbianism and stuttering, and ran to 300 personality types.[22]

As a young profession in the 1940's and 50's psychiatry fostered a belief in 'happiness pills' and forensic psychiatry, with theoretical justification from learning theory and psychoanalysis. Alcoholism was claimed as an area of competence and behaviour modification techniques were introduced in treatment. As it became clear that there was no tablet that could change personality, and as alcoholics staunchly refused to benefit from the cures offered to them, and because the faith in the efficacy of psychoanalysis was never strong, psychiatrists reversed their claim to competence and decided that these people were not mentally ill. People who suffer from alcoholism have represented enormous difficulties in integration into a medical classificatory system given that the responsibility for their behaviour has been increasingly viewed as their own.

Modern-day psychiatrists have inherited these over-ambitious claims to competence and have sought to jettison difficult areas of responsibility. At the same time, the field of psychogeriatrics has become a new speciality and rehabilitation another area of created experise encouraged by the government policy to return patients to the community.

At the same time as psychiatry was expanding its area of expertise, the establishment of the National Health Service entitled all to free and equal access to a doctor. However, the mediation of the state has guaranteed the right to service but not the manner of delivery. For the individual, the N.H.S. has established his right to define himself as ill which has been described as 'a reification of problems within the body of the patient from social to physical'.[23]

When dealing with patients whose difficulties are as much social as natural, general practitioners are faced with a number of alternatives. They may seek to change their patients' view of illness; this, however is a time-consuming process. A speedier solution is the prescription of minor tranquillisers but good medical practice is now seen as resistance to patients' demands for such a solution. A third alternative is referral to the psychiatric services and psychiatry has acted as a residual category in medicine. In the past, its eagerness to take on new areas of responsibility has made it receptive to the demands of people for a medical solution.

The degree of conflict and contradiction between society's expectations and the profession's ideology is determined by the extent to which the two can be satisfactorily enmeshed. On the one hand, there are psychiatrists who are faced with the consequences of their past enthusiasm to medicalise and take responsibility for new areas of behaviour. On the other hand, there is a receptive audience of potential patients who are eager to enjoy the benefits of the sick role.

The Deserving and Undeserving

Medical decisions are presented as neutral affairs of 'natural science'. Diagnostic activity mystifies such decision-making by allowing the display of abstract and specialised knowledge. In the field of mental illness, these methods camouflage the fact that judgements are being made about everyday behaviour. It is Szasz's argument that psychiatry has been enlisted by society to cloak unpleasant decisions in an aura of scientific objectivity and respectability.[24]

Scheff depicts mental illness as a residual category containing diverse kinds of behaviour that are lumped together into an explicit label for the convenience of society.[25] This picture has been substantiated in this study with a wide range of problem behaviours being displayed by patients. The problem for the psychiatrist is how to organise this diversity of behaviours into an identifiable and treatable group. How this is done is to divide patients into two groups which are here described as deserving and undeserving. The deserving group displays behaviour that can be fitted into a psychiatric classification and which may be amenable to treatment. They receive the approval of staff as 'genuinely mentally ill'.

Those not so accredited are a residual group and are here described as undeserving. Their behaviour does not fit into a medical model of mental illness and is not likely to be changed by treatment. They are often described in pejorative terms as malingering, demanding, attention-seeking and manipulating. The fact that these people are patients is linked to their raised expectations of medicine and their demands for treatment.

There are a number of alternatives available to psychiatrists in accommodating themselves to this undeserving group. The psychiatrist may go on the offensive and seek to keep such patients out of hospital. This may be done by a blacklist of those patients not to be admitted. If in hospital, they may be encouraged to discharge themselves against medical advice by such methods as stopping medication or transfer to an uncomfortable hospital back ward.

A second alternative for the psychiatrist is to pass on responsibility for such patients to para-medical staff within the hospital. This responsibility is seen as of a lower-order importance.[26] A third alternative for the psychiatrist is to award a diagnosis of 'genuinely mentally ill' to a previously 'undeserving' case thus transferring him into the deserving category. At the same time, the patient's status is legitimised to the extent that other staff support the psychiatrist's judgement. The change in the reasoning process is depicted below.

Medical Model
SYMPTOMS DIAGNOSIS TREATMENT

Pragmatic
DIAGNOSIS SYMPTOMS TREATMENT

Labelling may be used in a pragmatic way to justify a particular course of action and a recent feature of diagnostic activity has been movement between the two statuses of deserving and undeserving. When patients move between psychiatrists there is more likelihood of such delabelling as doctors review each others' decision-making. Changes in status also occur as patient career develops and when someone returns regularly to hospital the frequency of hospitalisaion may be used to justify a deserving label.

With high demand for the benefits of the sick role, some doctors resort to standards of fair play and act rather like a referee ensuring that as many people as possible have a chance to be admitted to hospital. There are obvious difficulties in maintaining the purity of the classificatory model and the psychiatrist may well become disillusioned. To the envy of hospital doctors G.P.'s cream off the most straightforward cases leaving hospital staff with the more difficult, both desrving and undeserving. Cynicism or the development of interests such as research are some of the ways doctors may cope with the disappointments of the medical model not meeting their expectations of it.

The Management of Conflict

The moral component of psychiatrists' decision-making is revealed in decisions about hospital treatment or police involvement. Szasz argues that the intervention of psychiatry in matters of right and wrong has obscured the differences between madness and badness and has created a confusion amongst members of society about matters of morality.[27] However, societal values and attitudes still determine the extent to which behaviour can be labelled as illness in the courtroom. If a crime has outraged public opinion it is likely that punishment will be demanded and meted out, in spite of any amount of expert psychiatric opinion of insanity.[28]

The rules that govern psychiatrists' behaviour in this respect are largely pragmatic. A crucial variable is the strength of patient status; if a person who has offended has a previous history of admissions then it is common for a psychiatric opinion to be requested. Indeed, the police are as likely to seek hospitalisation rather than court action in order to end their involvement. Whether the psychiatrist intervenes actively on the patient's behalf will depend on his being a deserving case.

If, however, a patient, who is at the beginning of a patient career, and who does not belong to the category of 'genuinely mentally ill', is in trouble with the police then he may be quickly discharged to prevent his achieving the ascribed status of psychiatric patient. Once the psychiatrist has assumed responsibility or had it thrust upon him, then the psychiatric label sticks on the labelled individual for the convenience of the courts who will have a ready means of disposal. Decisions that are taken for tactical reasons serve to redefine the moral territory between 'mad and bad'. Such boundaries are fluid and vary from case to case, which coupled with the fluidity of public opinion can result in bewilderment and inconsistency.

The boundaries of morality are also enforced in a less obvious way by psychiatrists in their discrimination between the deserving and undeserving. The implication of relabelling from deserving to undeserving is that the individual is again responsible for his actions. and further rule-breaking should be dealt with by the police. Whilst the psychiatrist may be able to reverse his decisions, it is not so straightforward for those emotionally involved, not least the patient. The situation is dramatically portrayed in the example of one patient who having been removed from hospital by the police proceeded to jump back in through the window. The outcome in such cases will be determined by the relative bargaining strengths of the interested parties - patient, family, psychiatrist and other agencies.

The Psychiatrist-Patient Relationship

The doctor-patient relationship in the National Health Service has been described as one dominated by the doctor who offers the minimum amount of information to the patient and who has little interest in the patient's point of view.[29] Most G.P.s are faced with full waiting rooms and seek to control consultations as tightly as possible.[30] Patients who insist on asking questions about diagnosis and treatment may be regarded as 'difficult'. This is because they take up more time and call into question the doctor as expert. There is a 'ritual' aspect to medical consultation which is characterised by an impersonality and politeness in which the patient is ascribed a reputable character and the doctor does not expect his judgement to be questioned. These aspects of medical consultation in the N.H.S. have been summed up in the phrase 'medical gentility'.[31]

The psychiatrist-patient relationship contains these features but it also has particular characteristics. The interview is of central importance in psychiatry. In general medicine the doctor can rely more on scientific procedures such as X-rays, and laboratory tests to elicit symptoms. The psychiatrist too sends for laboratory tests, E.E.G.'s (electroencaphalograms to measure brain waves) at an early stage in medical consultation. But it is the interview which provides the opportunity to evoke an array of statements - a display of talk on which the psychiatrist can base a therapeutic description of the patient's mind. Questions are not requests for information so much as an attempt to elicit material that can be categorised into symptomatology.

The psychiatrist may hope to maintain an aura of 'medical gentility' about his interaction with patients in order to neutralise areas of conflict. But aggressive behaviour is one of the frequent behaviours preceding hospitalisation and patients may need to be compulsory detained. Further, some patients believe they are not ill and that they are the victims of a mistake or persecution. All these characteristics make for a difficult case for treatment.

Except in organic conditions, such as a brain tumour, the term mental illness does not refer to some determinable underlying state or condition of the body. Rather, it involves judgements about beliefs and conduct which are partly based on the psychiatrist's own notion of adequate performance.[32] Abnormal behaviour is judged against previous behaviour; for instance, religious delusions are compared with the individual's previous level of religiosity. Information about previous behaviour has to be gleaned from the patient's family and is not usually immediately available, and decisions are taken in the interim on the basis of the psychiatrist's own 'rules of thumb'.

It is important to emphasise the everyday nature of the material upon which judgements are made. Topics range from pigeon racing to joinery, and inevitably the psychiatrist may have little precise knowledge and less experience. The everyday nature of a psychiatric interview is shown in this excerpt.

> Patient: "I'm going to change the carpet, move the bannister, decorate the house, give the carpet to the neighbours. Get a green one - I like green. Buy a companion set. Get velvet wallpaper - £15 a roll...."

The patient's description of her plans is interpreted by the psychiatrist as evidence of grandiose ideas, a symptom of hypomania. The terms are technical but the reasoning is commom sense theorising. Another example is the question to the patient, 'do you burn the pots?' in order to establish her level of disorientation. In such theorising, any discrepancy between professional notions of performance and wider notions of adequate performance are crucial in determining the relationship between psychiatry and society.

Such decision-making is influenced by the context in which behaviour occurs; the place of performance is a fundamental part of the evidence.[33] For the psychiatrist the fact that a person is talking in this particular way and is in hospital will influence the way he judges that behaviour. One of the working rules for all hospital staff in order to make work meaningful, is that a person's presence in hospital, de facto, indicates that his performance prior to admission has been causing problems for others. The psychiatrist is obliged to take in good faith the actions of others in getting the person into hospital.

Goffman has described the ways in which persons are seduced into hospital by their families.[34] Once in hospital, as patients they are also seduced into revealing their thoughts, beliefs and biography. This is encouraged by a mileau which is friendly, casual, and overtly unthreatening. Staff call patients by their first names and intrude into previously private and personal areas of behaviour in a non-commital and casual manner. Patients return to their own clothes, fraternise as they wish, smoke and watch television as they want, and the majority take their tablets and stay in hospital till their doctor discharges them.

The nature of the doctor-patient relationship is similar, although characterised by more formality. The use of formal names to patients encourages in return the use of the title 'doctor'. The patient is to trust and confide in his doctor; complaints are listened to and passed on to staff. In such ways the doctor puts across the message 'I'm on your side' and 'I'm here to help you'.

The questions posed by the psychiatrist are essentially designed to elicit information about the patient's conduct and thoughts. Interaction in our society is usually based on a set of understandings by both parties about what is to take place: 'rules of the game'.[35] In the psychiatrist-patient relationship one party, the patient, may be somewhat unclear about what is expected. The psychiatrist is concerned to avoid antagonism and phrases his questions in a bland way. For example, 'how's your thinking?': 'what was all that about?' (referring to an episode of disturbing behaviour); these are questions that contain no evaluative component to convey how the questioner views the behaviour of the respondent. No clues are given as to how to reply. The psychiatrist does not use the term suicide with all its pejorative connotations but 'did you ever think of ending it all?'

These questions are designed to elicit talk, that on inspection will reveal possibilities for categorising the talker's troubles. It is possible that the talker might sabotage the process by refusing to answer or by reinterpreting the question. In one of my own interviews the question 'How did you come to be in hospital?' was answered with 'By taxi'. Such literal interpretations are evidence of misinterpretation, themselves items for categorisation. One of the textbook methods for elucidating 'disordered thought' is to ask the patient to interpret a well-known proverb. When this question is asked, no reason is given for asking it and neither is one usually requested.

Steps in Decision Making

The ways that psychiatrists make decisions are not markedly different from other occupational groups operating in areas of uncertainty.[36] There are four broad steps in the decision-making process. In the first place, alternatives are ruled out. The fact of being in psychiatric hospital almost certainly means a psychiatric diagnosis. Within the system of categorisation, there are clear opportunities to attach particular descriptions that contain moral implications. The diagnosis of personality disorder carries with it the message that this patient cannot be cured, that his behaviour cannot be changed and that he should be discouraged from being in hospital because he then has 'the excuse' that he is ill. On the other hand, the 'genuinely mentally ill', the psychotic group, are desired for the opportunity to use specialised knowledge, to diagnose and to treat. The psychiatrist will be more positive about the treatment of such 'interesting cases' and be less willing to relinquish involvement.

The second step is the collection of evidence to decide between deserving and undeserving. What is crucial is whether such evidence is collected before or after the decision has been made. Every occupational group develops intuition and psychiatrists are no different in this respect. Having a gut feeling that something is wrong with a patient is 'evidence' justified by experience. Ward staff sometimes talk of someone being 'a bit schizophrenic' by the look in their eyes. More formal methods of collecting evidence include from the patient by the methods described above, from other staff in the hospital and from the patients's family. A biography of the patient is constructed and interpreted from the present status of the person as a psychiatric patient. Particular incidents and behaviours are emphasised which support the diagnosis of mental illness. It is the argument of Movahedi that such information can be selected from all our biographies.[37] Staff observe the patient on the ward and describe and define behaviour into a particular identity which becomes an established image. What exists in abundance on a psychiatric ward is information and pieces of information are in a perpetual state of motion between staff members and disciplines.

The third step is the construction of an explanatory model. For example, in order to diagnose schizophrenia, the following items of behaviour are identified from the patient's behaviour: listening to 'voices' (aural hallucination), being suspicious of people (paranoia), having difficulty in expressing ideas (thought blocking), having unusual beliefs about the situation which cannot be challenged (delusional systems), feeling emotions inappropiate to the stimulii (incongruity of affect), and feeling that everything has a direct effect on oneself (ideas of reference). These are the positive symptoms of schizophrenia. Other items of behaviour which are termed the negative symptoms of the condition include: failure to fulfill potential according to background (social drift), solitariness (withdrawal), and apathy and laziness (psychomotor retardation). When all of these symptoms are reported in a biography then the diagnosis of schizophrenia is a likely result.

Finally, psychiatrists develop 'on the job' practices to accomplish their task. These methods are pragmatic in nature, are developed over time, and form the content of their daily activity. For example, prepatients at home are visited in the morning when the symptoms of depression are more evident than later in the day. When looking for evidence of disturbed thinking, questions are asked about T.V. watching and radio listening since beliefs of thoughts being controlled are often connected with these appliances. Such characteristics of psychiatrists at work can be usefully itemised into 'rules of thumb' and are now described.

Rules of Thumb for Psychiatrists

Psychiatry shares a number of characteristics with other areas of medical activity. Psychiatrists are required to take decisions of great magnitude, in situations of uncertainty within the limits of their technical knowledge. Doctors must have a belief in the soundness of their ideas and the efficiency of their procedures. This has been described as 'optimistic bias'.[38] They have a predilection to activity, the medical ethos being one of intervention in a positive way through treatment. In the search for suitable responses, there is a tendency to seize on new treatments which are hailed as breakthroughs but are in the nature of fads, that go in and out of fashion.

The doctor-patient relationship is, of course, a two-way process. The doctor faces the demands of patients to do something and may well treat or admit to hospital in acquiescence. He is then required to diagnose on the basis of a discovered symptomatology. Medicine is no different from other occupations in this respect: there are two worlds, the theoretical and the practical. There is feedback between these two worlds. In the theoretical world, a classificatory system of mental illness as separate entities is rigidly adhered to. In the practical world, it is recognised that mental illness exists along a continuum. By such pragmatic idealism do psychiatrists accomplish some kind of order in their activity.

One method of work is to diagnose according to response to treatment: if a patient improves after a course of E.C.T. then a diagnosis of depression is confirmed. Whilst theorists might frown at such unscientific activity, such methods are common throughout medicine.[39] Doctors are reluctant to begin with a severe diagnosis, understandably not wishing to disturb a patient unnecessarily. In psychiatry, patient career and diagnosis go hand-in-hand; first admissions are defined as psychotic episode, periodic readmissions becomes a defining characteristic of schizophrenia.

The adverse effects of labelling discourage early diagnosis of several mental illnesses. There is a reluctance for psychiatrists, however, to share diagnosis of severe mental illness with patient and family for a number of reasons. One reason is to avoid frightening the patient's caretakers into abandoning him. Contemporary philosophy in psychiatry is community orientated and this has made psychiatrists very sensitive to the question of disposal.

The implications of medical decisions are far-reaching, and the psychiatrist feels his responsibilities. The establishment of the National Health Service has demonstrated the political power of those who make up its patients. The financial interests and prestige of the medical profession are under political management to this degree and doctors are sensitive not to antagonise a public who is the consumer of their services. Their sensitivity is heightened by their fears of litigation should they be found incompetent or guilty of malpractice. Because of these factors doctors may adopt a policy of 'safety first' and allow what they might otherwise regard as inappropiate admissions. If such patients subsequently leave hospital against medical advice doctors may then be seen to have offered help which has been rejected.

Summary

This chapter has been concerned to describe the values and the rules (which are determined by the interplay of values) which govern the ways in which psychiatrists use the concept of mental illness. The important identified variables are their professional ideology and the societal expectations of them. The activity of the psychiatrist crystallises around several moral issues; he navigates his way through this moral quagmire with the assistance of his rules of thumb. He is in charge of the marriage of a variety of standpoints into a systematic approach. This approach should also be professionally rewarding for him, fulfilling the expectations of his professional ideology.

The concept 'dirty work' has been identified to describe an area of an occupation where one is compelled to play a role which 'one thinks one ought to be a little morally ashamed'.[40] All occupations have some kind of dirty work and there are a number of ways of accommodating it. Dignifying rationalisations serve to elevate such work by emphasising its contribution to other long term goals. The sacrifice of short term means for long term goals is one such rationalisation.[41] Another accommodation is to transform or scale down occupational goals. The problem here for psychiatrists is that they subscribe to occupational goals that belong to a different, albeit a parent, profession. Occupational goals for medicine are often over-ambitious for psychiatry. The problems that people bring into psychiatric hospital are sometimes intractable. They may abate, perhaps return and even increase. The whole of psychiatry becomes something of an area of necessary but 'dirty work' for practitioners who subscribe to the occupational ideology of medicine.

Notes

1. Goffman, E. (1961) *Asylums*, Harmondsworth.
2. Rosenham, D. (1973) 'On being Sane in Insane Places'. *Science*, Jan 1973, pp. 250-58. Eight researchers reported symptoms of schizophrenia to gain entry to a psychiatric hospital, and then behaved normally in hospital; they were uniformly diagnosed schizophrenic and kept for varying periods from seven to fifty two days.
3. Bastide, R. (1972) *The Sociology of Mental Disorder*, London.
4. The 1986 Mental Health Order is a good example of this change in attitude. The Order prevents the compulsory admission of people diagnosed as having a personality disorder, or suffering from alcoholism.
5. Becker, H. (1961) *Boys in White*, Chicago. This is a sociological study of medical school, and the development of 'pragmatic idealism'.
6. Johnson, T. (1972) *Professions and Power*, Essex; see Chapter 6.
7. Parsons, T. (1951) *The Social System*, New York. See Chapt. 10 in which the author lists four mechanisms of control: universalistic, functionally specific, affectively neutral and collectively-oriented. With regard to functionally-specific this control no longer operates as doctors as the 'new clergy' pronounce on all manner of moral issues.
8. For example, the symptoms of endogenous depression are early morning wakening, loss of weight and appetite, feelings of hopelessness, delusions of guilt, nihilistic delusions, and suicidal ideas.
9. Kraepelin, E., was the founding father of the classificatory system (1855-1926).
10. Armor, D. and Klerman, G. (1969) 'Psychiatric Treatment Orientations and Professional Ideology', *Journal of Health and Social Behaviour*, 9, pp. 243-55.
11. Henrey, W., Simms, J. and Spray, S. (1971) The Fifth Profession, San Francisco.
12. Taylor, J. (1965) 'The Organisation of Physicians' Attitudes towards the Emotionally Disturbed Patient', *Journal of Health and Social Behaviour*, 6, pp. 99-104.

13. Redlich, F., Hollingshead, A. and Ballis, E. (1955) 'Social Class Differences in Attitudes towards Psychiatry'. *American Journal of Orthopsychiatry*, 25, pp. 60-70. The researchers found that therapists generally disapproved of the behaviour patterns of lower class patients, their sexual mores, low verbal intelligence, and dependency. Therapists failed to understand their values and were frustrated by the failure to achieve therapeutic gains. These feelings were especially marked for the upwardly mobile therapists.
14. Bean, P. (1980) *Compulsory Admissions to Mental Hospital*, London. The author accompanied eight psychiatrists on emergency visits to patients' homes and studied their decision-making with regard to compulsory admission.
15. Beck, A. (1962) 'Reliability of Psychiatric Diagnoses: A Study of Consistency of Clinical Judgements and Ratings', *American Journal of Psychiatry*, 119, pp. 351-7. The subjective element in such judgements is underlined by the unreliability of diagnoses between psychiatrists. Beck found an overall agreement between four psychiatrists of under 54 per cent. An example of cultural differences in the present research is the description of wearing a black T-short under a white shirt as bizarre and hence a symptom of illness.
16. Laing, R. and Esterson, A. (1964) *Sanity, Madness and the Family*, London.
17. Leff, J. and Vaughan, C. (1981) 'The Role of Maintenance Therapy and Relatives' Expressed Emotion in Relapse in Schizophrenics'. *British Journal of Psychiatry*, 139, pp. 102-4.
18. Kuhn, T. (1962) *The Structure of Scientific Revolution*, Chicago. Kuhn describes a 'paradigm clash' when a variety of fundamentally different viewpoints are competing for ascendancy. He suggests this is a distinct stage in the development of fields of scientific enquiry.
19. Armor, D. and Klerman, G. (1969) op cit. It seems that psychoanalysts frequently combine drugs with psychotherapy in their practice.
20. Foucault, M. (1965) *Madness and Civilisation: A History of Insanity in the Age of Reason*, London.
21. Illich, I. (1976) *Limits to Medicine*, London. He describes three types of iatrogenic disease:
1) Clinical - where remedies, physicians or hospitals are the sickening agents;
2) Social - where medical practice sponsors sickness by reinforcing a morbid society;
3) Cultural - an expropiation of health by which the health of people is denied.
22. World Health Organisation (1979) *Glossary of Mental Disorders.*
23. Strong, P. (1979) *The Ceremonial Orders of the Clinic.*
24. Szasz, T. (1972) *The Manufacture of Madness*, London, Chapt. 11 'Since psychiatry deals with personal and social conduct, and such cannot be described or evaluated without anchoring it in a matrix of values, there is nothing to confuse between rules of mental health and rules of mortality. They are one and the same'.
25. Scheff, T. (1966) *Being Mentally Ill*, London.

26. Johnson, T. (1975) op. cit. In the National Health Service auxiliary health professionals are defined by statute as 'professions supplementary to medicine', see p. 58.
27. Szasz, T. op cit. to quote: 'By being considered simultaneously a malefactor (as mad) like the criminal and a victim (as sick) like the sick patient, the mental patient obliterates the distinction bewteen criminal and non-criminal, guilty and innocent'.
28. A recent example is Peter Sutcliffe, 'the Yorkshire Ripper', first sent to prison against psychiatric recommendations, now in Broadmoor.
29. Stimson and Webb, J. (1975) *Going to see the Doctor*, London.
30. Ibid. It has been found that the average length of consultation with a G.P. is 6 - 15 minutes.
31. Strong, P. op. cit.
32. Coulter, G. (1973) *Approaches to Insanity*, London. He states: 'psychiatric practices are bound up with the pragmatics of living and the objectivity of psychiatric judgements is more a matter of reasonableness and necessary precautions in specific cases than of operating according to universal, culture-neutral principles and procedures'.
33. Goffman, E. (1971) *Relations in Public*, London. Appendix, 'The Insanity of Place'. Goffman describes manic behaviour in terms of its effects on the place where it occurs.
34. Goffman, E. (1960) op. cit.
35. Blum, A. 'The Sociology of Mental Illness' in Douglas, J. (1970) *Deviance and Respectability - The Social Construction of Moral Meanings*, New York. Blum's approach contains the essence of the ethnomethodological approach.
36. Atkinson, M. (1982) *Discovering Suicide - Studies in the Social Organisation of Sudden Death*, London. The author describes a similar process of decision-making by coroners investigating sudden death.
37. Movahedi, S. (1975) 'Loading the Dice in Favour of Madness' *Journal of Health and Social Behaviour*, 16, pp. 192-7. The author asked his students to compile their biographies emphasising their bleak experiences. Only 7 per cent of biographies could not be classified as psychiatrically disturbed.
38. Parsons, T. (1951) op. cit.
39. White, K. 'Evaluation of Medical Education and Health Care', in *Community Medicine, Teaching and Health Care* eds, Lathan, W. and Newberry, A. (1970) New York.
    It has been estimated that as much as 50 per cent of ambulatory complaints do not fit into the International Disease Classification.
40. Emerson, R. and Pollner, M. (1976) 'Dirty Work Designations: Their Features and Consequences in a Psychiatric Setting'. *Social Problems*. 23. pp. 243-54. The authors examined the work of a community mental health team and utilised Everett Hughes's concept of dirty work to describe their attitude to hospitalising patients against their will.
41. Bean, P. (1980) op. cit.

11 Conclusion

In this research study, I have found that psychiatric hospitalisation is a very complicated social process in which there is no straightforward relationship between illness and hospitalisation. Anyone who reads this study will find it hard to accept the view that people are hospitalised because they are iller than those who are not hospitalised. Individuals suffer sickness, but how patient career develops can only be understood in terms of the activities of various groups studied. The study of the social construction of mental illness requires the consideration of the attitudes and activities of those personally and professionally involved.

It can be seen that the social process of psychiatric hospitalisation is necessarily complex as it involves the interaction between many factors which may operate sometimes in opposing directions and feedback their effects upon each other. This complexity makes conceptualisation difficult. Any analysis of social activity requires a proposed model which will broadly represent the actuality, and which will organise disparate acts and events into a coherent whole. However, such are the complexity of forces in the process of psychiatric hospitalisation, so various are the contingencies that operate, and the alternative outcomes available, that ending up in psychiatric hospital may almost seem a fortuitous event. Nevertheless, the analysis of the patient sample did produce a picture of a deprived group of people in terms of social disintegration, employment, income and housing. Their common characteristics were that they were working class, lived alone, and more likely to be unmarried and female.

A number of competing explanations were outlined, along with the various difficulties of substantiating the superiority of one theoretical approach over another. Having started from the point of hospitalisation it was not possible to answer the qustion of social causation. As a single researcher it was quite impossible for me, with limited time and resources, to test out such theories. Rather, my attention was focused on the routes that people followed to hospital and the activities of the various groups involved.

Working part-time, I have only been able to take this study so far. It is necessarily preliminary in its broad sketch of the social process of psychiatric hospitalisation. There is scope for more detailed research into particular areas such as family interaction and the negotiation of conflict. A follow-up study would be useful to establish how far being mentally ill has become a master status or, to what extent, it has been possible to invoke other labels. A complementary study of 'routes out of hospital' would now seem necessary to further illuminate the dynamics of hospitalisation. The labelling approach to deviance generally has failed to address this question of how people get delabelled.

I have sought to describe each labelling group on the route to psychiatric hospitalisation. The various activities, ideologies and definitions of personal and professional labellers are outlined, along with the institutional provision and contingencies, to describe a broad conceptualisation of the social process of psychiatric hospitalisation.

The story of psychiatric hospitalisation is now summarised. An extreme labelling approach, which neglects initial behaviour, and supposes that only labelling and the responses to it are important, has not been adopted in this research. Rather it has been recognised that how people behave is relevant. Many of the people labelled mentally ill do behave in strange ways which distress their families. Patient career develops from the labelling of outsiders and the interaction of the patient with his labellers. How and when labelling takes place is explained by a whole series of contingencies which provide many ways of arriving at the same outcome.

When an aberrant act occurs it may be viewed in a number of ways by the family. The perpetrator, himself, may recognise his action as a symptom of illness and in this case automatic referral to a doctor will probably follow. However, the family's attitude becomes crucial when the act is denied by the individual. The family may be prepared to go along with this interpretation and label behaviour as eccentric or seek to normalise it by the use of 'rational' explanations in terms of stress or other extrinsic factors. Should the family follow this path they will have to mobilise alternatives definitions of deviance. These will include, on the one hand, acceptance of behaviour as a 'burden' and, on the other hand, defining it as wilful and labelling the perpetrator as a miscreant.

The extent to which behaviour is defined as acceptable or unacceptable is likely to be determined not only by its extremity but also by its visibility. Clearly, when someone acts in a bizarre way in a public place it is considerably more difficult to deny such behaviour than if it had been witnessed either by a small number of family or completely hidden in private. The larger the number of different roles an individual performs, the more he is under public observation. Public behaviour is likely to draw the attention of friends, neighbours and, in more extreme cases, social agencies such as the police. All these witnesses will make their own decisions as to the nature of the behaviour. They, too, may be sympathetic and regard it as the result of misfortune or perhaps as being of religious significance. If the police do not accept an illness defintion then they are more likely to criminalise behaviour and social workers will be concerned to assess the degree of risk.

Different families will accept different levels of behaviour. The extent to which a family will continue to accept unusual behaviour, given its range and visibility, will be determined by their level of tolerance. Family tolerance may be influenced by the importance of the individual to the family network and by wider attitudinal factors. If a mother is crucial to the survival of a family and for the care of young children, a definition of behaviour which results in hospitalisation is likely to be avoided for as long as possible. Excesses of behaviour may well be tolerated to a much greater degree from such an important family member than from someone on the family periphery with few vital functions. Tolerance may stem from a more fatalistic attitude towards hardship which explains difficulties as bad luck, an attitude more frequently found in the lower social classes. The level of expectations is also important; those with lower expectations are more likely to accept swings in behaviour.

Admission may be delayed when a family hold a negative attitude towards mental illness. Such an attitude may be the result of the experience of hospital incarceration within the sub-culture. It may also be prompted by a fear of the stigmatising consequences of the mental illness label. In both cases, the family are more likely to use a physical illness explanation which does not carry such stigma. Once the family has interpreted behaviour as evidence of mental illness then it may be more ready to resort to such a label in the future. Familiarity with psychiatric staff and hospital may overcome stigma so that the hospital is perceived as a ready source of help. The mental illness label can become a master status for the individual with all his acts being judged in reference to it.

Not only is attitude to mental illness important but the family will also be influenced by the category of mental illness in which their relative has been placed. The family may repond more favourably to a diagnosis, such as senile dementia caused by hardening of the arteries in the brain, that is similar to physical illness. Such a diagnosis does not blame the individual for his circumstances but fully justifies entry to the sick role and the enjoyment of his family's attention. A diagnosis of personality disorder, however, carries a moral implication that the individual is, in some sense, in control of and responsible for his behaviour. His family are then more likely to find his behaviour unacceptable and describe it in perjorative terms such as malingering or manipulating.

The family reaction is further influenced by the expected course of the condition. Roles have to be revised following admission and again renegotiated after recovery and return home. A single episode, successfully treated followed by full recovery would cause minimal family disruption and would be the preferred outcome. However, this is unlikely given that mental illness is very often recurring and difficult to treat.

Medical contingencies also play a large part in determining the likelihood of hospitalisation. These contingencies include the doctor's attitude towards mental illness and his willingness to use the mental illness label. He too may resort to alternative explanations and use the mental illness label only as a last resort when persuaded by family pressure or threats to abandon the individual. The reluctant doctor may be left with few alternatives but hospitalisation. Another medical contingency is the time of doctor's visit as clearly, options are limited at night. The most important determinant of outcome is, however, availability of hospital beds, this overrides all other considerations. Scarcity of beds means that, regardless of the nature of behaviour and the family level of enlightenment, the family will have to find alternative solutions.

The movement to hospital has four components. In the first place, there is a social movement from one set of roles to another. In the second place, each set of roles is accompanied by a new status which is determined by the act of labelling. In the third place, there is an ideological movement from one set of attitudes to another as the individual and significant others respond to the label. Finally, there is a geographical movement from one place to another into hospital.

This movement is not so much linear as a downward spiral as the individual takes on a stigmatised status with long-term consequences for self-esteem, social integration, and functioning. It has been seen that what takes place is not usually a cataclysmic occurrence, although the final act of hospitalisation may be quite dramatic. It is rather a gradual process of interpretation and re-interpretation of a succession of minor events and acts of behaviour by significant others. This is a process of action and reaction which contains a feedback effect on the behaviour in question.

The geographical movement is described in the diagram 'Pathways to Hospital' which also shows the chief agents on each route who act as both labellers and gatekeepers to determine hospitalisation. The separate components of routes, dimensions and labels are combined into a model that portrays the movement to hospital as circular and downward. This model seeks to include the feedback effects between labeller and labellee, label and self-definition, attitude and response, labelling and future attitude, and contingency and outcome.

The social process of psychiatric hospitalisation can truly be seen as multi-dimensional. It is hoped that the present research has done something to unravel the major factors in operation and, by so doing, has helped to clarify and illuminate what actually happens.

Diagram Two; Pathways to Hospital

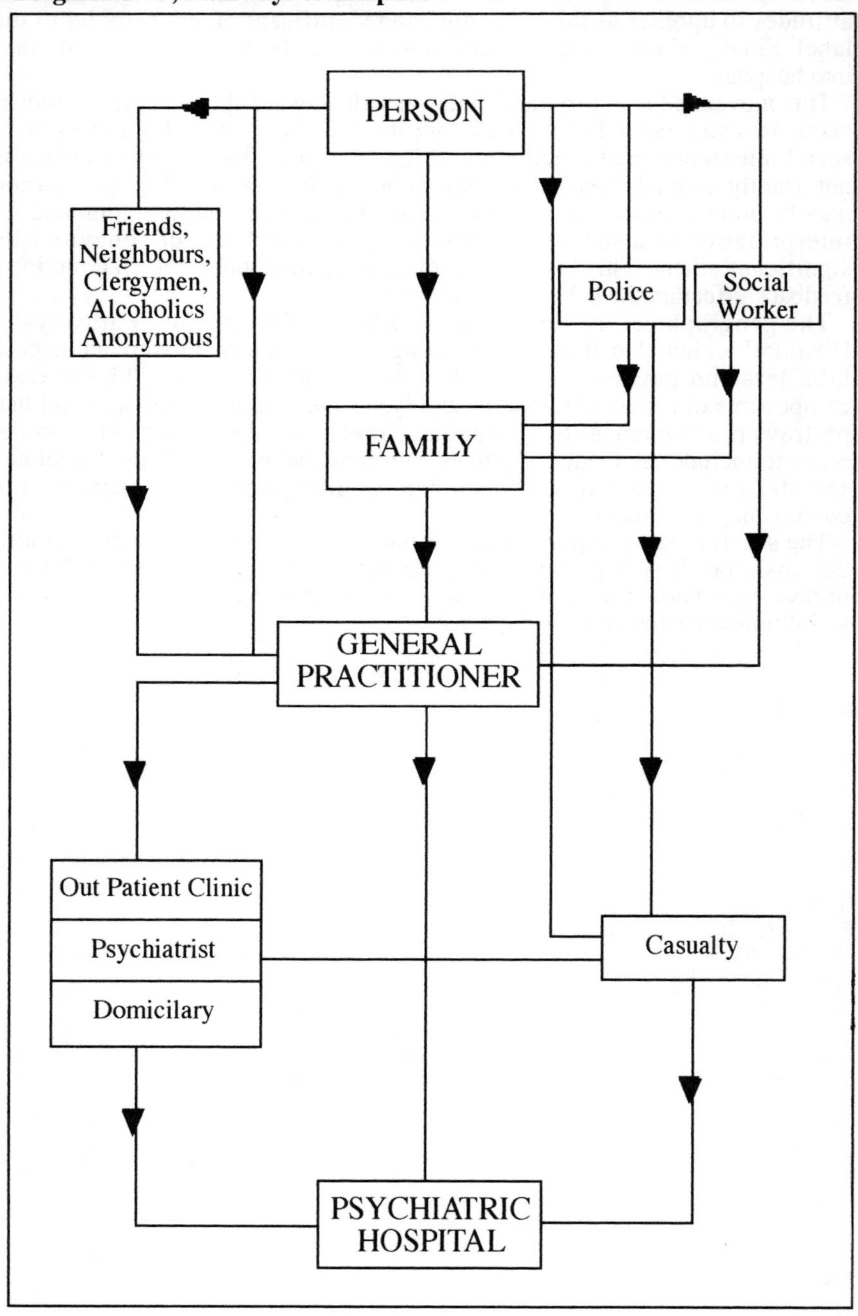

Appendices

Appendix 11.1

Numbers, Social Class, Previous Admissions and Diagnoses of District Patients entering City Psychiatric Hospitals (1974 & 1981)

Hospital		No.	S.C.	Prev. Adm.	Diagnosis
A	1981	3	S.CII - 1		Psychoses- 2
			V - 2		Unknown - 1
	1974	8			
B	1981	2			Neuroses - 2
C	1981	20	II - 2	1st Adm- 5	Psychoses- 7
			III -13	1 -5 ' - 2	Alcoholic- 4
			IV - 1	6-10 ' - 5	Pers. Dis- 3
			V - 2	Over 10- 7	Neuroses - 3
					Organic - 2
	1974	36			

Appendix 11.2

Number, Social Class and Diagnoses of those entering Psychiatric Care in a General Hospital (1981)

Hospital	No.	Social Class	Diagnosis
General	94	S.C.I - 2	Psychoses- 44
		II - 9	Neuroses - 34
		III - 33	Pers Dis - 11
		IV - 15	Other - 11
		V - 17	
		Unknown - 18	

Appendix 11.3

Patient Social class of Formal Admissions

Social Class	Per cent of Formal Adms.	Per cent of Patient Sample
I	-	1
II	9	8
III	50	41
IV	32	37
V	9	12
TOTAL	100	100

Categories of Problem Behaviours for Family Referrers

Problem Behaviour	Number	Per cent
Thought Disordered	23	35
Aggressive/Disruptive	20	31
Self-destructive	22	34

Appendix 11.4

Patients referred by Relatives according to Relationship of Relative and Sex of Patient

Family Referrers and Sex of Patient

	No. of Admissions		
Relative	Sex of Patient		Total
	Male	Female	
Spouse	9	12	21
Children	1	10	11
Parents	8	7	15
Siblings	3	3	6
TOTAL	21	32	53